THE PAIN CODE

WALKING THROUGH THE MINEFIELD
OF THE HEALTH SYSTEM

BARBY INGLE

THE PAIN CODE

WALKING THROUGH THE MINEFIELD
OF THE HEALTH SYSTEM

BARBY INGLE

Copyright © 2012 Barby Ingle

BK Publishing

Editor: Julie Jasper

All rights reserved

ISBN: 0615680321

ISBN-13: 978-0615680323

THE PAIN CODE

WALKING THROUGH THE MINEFIELD
OF THE HEALTH SYSTEM

BARD INGLE

Introduction Page

Patients all over America have been struggling to get good healthcare for chronic conditions. These patients, including myself, are suffering the pitfalls of the healthcare system. The sufferers of poor healthcare range from the patient to their family, providers, and millions of taxpayers.

In most chronic care situations, we are not taught self-advocacy skills. So, we do not know our rights or responsibilities as a patient. For this terrible situation to stop it is going to take a combined effort on the part of many people but it starts with us becoming informed, proactive, and organized. Excellent, prevention programs, access to care, and learning the tools to take care of ourselves between appointments will go a long way towards ending this crisis in our society.

Barby teaches these advocacy skills to the reader, so you are better prepared as a patient. You must be prepared and organized for your situation to receive the best healthcare possible. The topics are covered in a straightforward, non-technical manner, which allows you to understand quickly the fundamental principles of walking through the minefield of the health system.

Melissa Lucero, Pain Patient, Mother, and Advocate

Table of Contents

PAIN IS AN EPIDEMIC.................................9

Types of Pain 14

Neuropathy Pain.................................17

Be Aware of Depression 17

BECOME AN EXPERT ON YOUR ILLNESS 25

A Bit About Neuropathy.................................28

Types of Nerves 35

Identifying Symptoms 36

Types of Neuropathy.................................38

IT PAYS TO ORGANIZE YOUR HEALTHCARE 43

Treatment Options.................................46

Alternative Treatment.................................70

Requesting Healthcare Records 78

FACING FINANCIAL CHALLENGES.................................97

Finding Housing 97

Keeping the Lights On 100

Water and Energy Assistance 103

DISABILITY RESOURCES.................................111

Supplemental Security Income (SSI).................................111

Medicare 112

Medicaid 115

Military Benefits 115

Other State Assistance Programs 116

Food Stamps 117

Handicap Passes 119

Bus Passes 123

Transportation to your doctor visits 123

INSURANCE *127*

Medical Insurance 130

Dental Insurance 140

Explanation of Benefits (EOB) 143

Military Health Coverage 144

Workers Compensation 146

Challenges with Insurance 151

REACH OUT *165*

Make it a Family Affair 167

Finding Community 169

Support Groups 172

CREATE YOUR OASIS *177*

Living Well With Chronic Pain 180

Self-Care & Coping Skills 185

DEDICATION *202*

1

PAIN IS AN EPIDEMIC

When it comes to living the best life you can every person has choices. There are even more choices for those who face a chronic care condition daily. It is important to find the right fit for you. The patient can either let the disease run them or sort through the system and take control of the disease. According to the Institute of Medicine's 2011 report, 116 million Americans live with a chronic care condition that causes pain. These are incredible numbers and breaks down to one in three Americans facing pain every day. If it is not you, then it is probably someone you know.

Coping with a chronic condition takes hope and self-awareness. You can make it through the toughest of situations. I know because if I can do it anyone can. I have been facing an autoimmune condition, Reflex Sympathetic Dystrophy for ten years now. Through my struggles and finding my way, I have gained knowledge that I am going to pass on to you. Your first goal should be getting a correct diagnosis. If you need to go to multiple doctors, take the time to do it now to help prevent your health deteriorating in the future. Each doctor has their specialty as well as treatment options with which they are comfortable. This does not always mean that it is the right thing for you or that another option will not work. If you are not comfortable with the ones offered by the current provider, find a doctor who you trust to try different treatment options.

Getting organized is very important. It will take work in the beginning but it gets easier as you go. You can also save yourself more pain and challenges down the road by being organized with your approach to treating your chronic medical issue. It can be very aggravating to deal with a kidney stone or torn ligament but at least there is an end in sight. You can get back to "normal life" once the stone passes or the bone break heals. Other conditions such as high blood pressure, heart failure, diabetes, lyme, multiple sclerosis, RSD, arthritis, osteoporosis, neuropathy, or other chronic conditions, can be more of a challenge for patients and usually last a lifetime. Take charge of your disease instead of letting it rule you. Some doctors, friends, and even family can say, "just live with it" or "get used to it". You are the one who lives with this chronic condition. You can learn to live with it or learn to manage life around the symptoms and problems, without losing yourself.

For the person in pain there is a loss of quality of life. This can be due to financial burdens, loss of social support, and often by depression, which occurs after the condition is developed. Depression can result in isolation, loss of self-esteem, and self worth.

In 2003, GlaxoSmithKline funded a study on "Chronic Care in America". Their goal was to study and improve the patient-physician interaction. There were 3,000 adults and 1,000 doctors who completed the study on living and coping with a chronic condition. Many of the patients in the study who believe they were successful in the management of their chronic condition saw it more as a "long-term" or "ongoing" challenge.[1] In other words, once you understand your condition may not be cured with short-term treatments you can then begin to comprehend that the management of your condition will be ongoing. This is a factor in determining your level of successful outcome.

It is important to recognize that we need support as patients. We need positive attitudes and that there will be life changes. Some will be easier, a matter of changing your diet or beginning a physical therapy routine. Others will be more difficult such as having to sever ties to a family member or friend who is hindering your recovery. We also need the support from our healthcare providers. But most of all, we need to recognize that we are responsible for ourselves and that successful treatment may result in necessary lifestyle changes that only we can provide to ourselves.

We all deserve to have our pain taken seriously. To have the pain managed instead of under-

---

[1] Harris Interactive, GlaxoSmithKline, Chronic Care in America; Improving the Patient Physician Interaction. Findings from a comprehensive survey in the US, 2003

treated, untreated, or over-treated is an important aspect of successful treatment. Pain must be managed effectively and in a timely manner. The underlying condition needs to be addressed while the pain is being managed. Do not assume that your doctor knows how to treat your pain. Every patient is different and doctors only know what they have been exposed to in their schooling and continuing education classes. For example, if they are a regular attendee at a pain education conference they may skip the class on multiple sclerosis or lyme because they have a greater interest in migraines. As a patient it is up to you to become the chief of staff of your medical team and make sure you have a strong team willing to help, learn, and treat you.

The spotlight can also be shown on the cost of pain in our society. Approximately 40 million Americans between ages 30 and 49, suffer from migraines. Chronic pain is a disease in itself. Until our system begins to recognize this as a whole and changes our practices to prevention verses treating the person after the fact could bring down the cost of care. For instance, teach children about good posture and body alignment and have them practice. This can help them keep the habit throughout adulthood, cutting down on back issues and conditions that lead to the need for chronic care.

We must be careful to get the proper healthcare professionals on our team. The goal is to receive effective relief and be able to organize and manage all aspects of life. Finding good healthcare and support systems will lower the number of hospital visits, amount of time spent in the hospital, unnecessary trips to the emergency room, repeated tests, and inadequate treatments. All of which contribute to the high costs of healthcare.

Types of Pain

Pain is categorized in two main categories. Acute pain is short-term pain, usually lasting weeks to 3 months. Chronic pain lasts longer than 3 months. Chronic pain is further broken down into somatic pain, visceral pain, and neuropathic pain. Pain is subjective, although using a common scale helps us rate it into a better understood ideal. Your pain is your pain and only you know what it is like to live with it day in and day out. Therefore, we need to trust that pain is what the person says it is.

Somatic Pain

- A common cause of somatic pain in people with spinal cord injury (SCI) is postsurgical pain from the surgical incision
- It is usually described as a dull or aching feeling
- Somatic pain is caused by the activation of pain receptors in either the body surface or musculoskeletal tissues
- Somatic pain is probably caused by a combination of factors, such as abnormalities that may have always been there, such as inflammation, repetitive trauma, excessive activity, vigorous stretching, contractions due to paralysis, spasticity, flabbiness, disuse, and misuse
- Somatic pain is usually aggravated by activity levels and relieved by rest
- Somatic pain, that is a complication of SCI, occurs with increased frequency in the

shoulders, hips, and hands, although it also occurs in the lower back and buttock

Visceral Pain

- Visceral pain is the pain we feel when our internal organs are damaged or injured and is by far the most common form of pain
- Visceral refers to the internal areas of the body that are enclosed in a cavity
- Visceral pain is caused by problems with internal organs, such as the stomach, kidney, gallbladder, urinary bladder, and intestines
- Visceral pain can also be caused by problems with abdominal muscles and the abdominal wall, such as spasms
- The problems of visceral pain include perforation, inflammation, and impaction or constipation which can cause associated symptoms such as nausea, fever, and pain
- Visceral pain is caused by the activation of pain receptors in the chest, abdomen or pelvic areas
- Visceral pain is vague and not well localized
- Visceral pain is usually described as pressure-like, deep squeezing, or dull

Neuropathy Pain

- Neuropathy Pain is caused by injury or malfunction to the spinal cord and/or peripheral nerves
- Neuropathy pain is scattered and occurs at the level or below the level of injury, most often in the legs, back, feet, thighs, and toes, although it can also occur in the buttocks, hips, upper back, arms, fingers, abdomen, and neck
- Neuropathy pain is typically described as a burning, tingling, shooting, stinging, or "pins and needles" sensation
- Some people also feel stabbing, electric, piercing, cutting, and drilling pain
- This type of pain usually occurs within days, weeks, or months of the injury and tends to occur in waves of frequency and intensity

Be Aware of Depression

Your mood does have a lot to do with the daily living you experience. Overwhelmingly, people with chronic diseases have depressive moods. Take this seriously, as depression can keep you from taking care of yourself. You cannot afford to let yourself fall into dark dreary moods. Be sure that no matter how you are feeling that you are following the goals set for your care. It is important to take the correct dose of medication at the correct time of each day.

Be sure to communicate with the healthcare professionals on your team. It may take a little effort to keep healthy habits when you are depressed. Learn the signs and ask for assistance when needed. Be sure to talk to your general doctor or cognitive therapist if you think you are depressed or heading in that direction. [2]

If you do not deal with the emotional aspects of your condition you may begin to isolate yourself from others, decrease mobility, and increase drug dependence. Pain is depressing, and a cycle begins where depression causes and intensifies pain and stress on your body. In a statement by the International Association for the Study of Pain, pain is defined as "an unpleasant sensory

---

[2] *Harvard Mental Health Letter. Sept 2004,*
www.health.harvard.edu/mental

or emotional experience associated with actual or potential tissue damage or described in terms of such damage." As patients, it can be hard to face the emotional aspects of pain, but it is important to look at the signs and be aware of them in your everyday life as a chronic pain patient. Remember, pain causes depression, not the other way around.

The nervous system works in a cyclic pattern. Your body communicates with your brain and then your brain sends back a message to your body. When the system is dysfunctioning, physical sensations including pain, are more likely to become our center of attention. Both pain and emotion is processed in the limbic region. When the normal process of the limbic system fails, pain is intensified along with sadness, hopelessness, anxiety, and stress. Pain alters the functioning of the nervous system and perpetuates itself and depression.

Techniques for Dealing With Depression
- Cognitive and behavioral therapies teach pain patients how to avoid fearful anticipation, banish discouraging thoughts, and adjust

everyday routines to ward off physical and emotional suffering

- Dealing with a chronic pain condition can slow the recovery from depression, specialists should treat both problems together
- Physical therapists provide exercises not only to break the vicious cycle of pain and immobility but also to help relieve depression
- Psychotherapy helps demoralized patients and their families tell their stories and describe the experience of pain in its relation to other problems in their lives
- Techniques, including progressive muscle relaxation, hypnosis, and meditation can be helpful in reducing pain levels and depression

Signs of Depression

Depression carries a high risk of suicide. Anybody who expresses suicidal thoughts or intentions should be taken very seriously. Do not hesitate to call your local suicide hotline immediately. Call 800-SUICIDE (800-784-2433) for immediate assistance. According to the

National Institute of Mental Health, symptoms of depression may include the following:[3]

- Difficulty concentrating, remembering details, and making decisions
- Fatigue and decreased energy
- Feelings of guilt, worthlessness, hopelessness and/or helplessness
- Insomnia, early-morning wakefulness, or excessive sleeping
- Irritability, restlessness
- Loss of interest in activities or hobbies once pleasurable, including sex
- Overeating or appetite loss
- Persistent aches or pains, headaches, cramps, or digestive problems that do not ease even with treatment
- Persistent sad, anxious, or "empty" feelings
- Thoughts of suicide, suicide attempt

Getting your depression under control can help you better focus on getting your chronic condition

[3] National Institute of Mental Health, NIMH Information Resource Center, 866-615-6464, NIH Publication No. 11-3561, Revised 2011 www.nimh.nih.gov/health/publications/depression/complete-index.html

under control. It will help lower pain levels as you learn to let go of anxiety and stress and develop a plan as well as goals. Work with your healthcare professionals to get past this challenge. Now that you undertand the different types of pain you can see how difficult it can be to get a proper diagnosis which can increase depression. With all of the challenges outlined in this chapter, it is not difficult to realize how pain became an epidemic.

Walking Through the Minefield of the Health System

2

BECOME AN EXPERT ON YOUR ILLNESS

Setting the expectation is important in challenging life situations. You can become an expert of your condition by doing research and keeping a journal. When you and the people around you understand your illness and treatment options, you will be better able to prepare and cope with the situation. Having knowledge of your illness from the research you keep in your journal can help you relieve fear, but the information needs to come from reliable sources. You can get condition-specific research from healthcare providers, the internet, support groups, local and national charities, and your pharmacist.

What do you do first – JUST ASK! If you do not understand something about your illness, treatment, side effects or outcomes of treatment, do your own research, ask your resources and find the answer before you make a decision that will affect your life. You must be comfortable with what you choose, otherwise, gather more information until you are okay with the decision you make. Keep asking until you understand the explanation. It is your right to know how you may be affected by any treatment option. Track your goals, questions, progress, physical, and emotional health, so that you can better talk to your healthcare providers. By keeping a journal, you can become an expert and begin to educate healthcare professionals, friends, and family about your condition.

Take care of your emotional well-being. This is as important as taking care of your physical well-being. Seeing a psychologist/psychiatrist is not something of which to be ashamed. Most people going through similar health challenges need support. Having a chronic illness is one of the most stressful situations you will ever face. Pay attention to your emotional balance. If you seem depressed, anxious, or feeling less secure in your situation, be sure to talk your feelings over with someone. This should be charted in your journal so that you can see patterns and expand your understanding. These patterns should be communicated with your support team, which should include family, friends, health, and mental health professionals.

I live by the motto, "Never give up, never give in." This can only be accomplished if you are responsible for yourself and your treatment choices. Get regular updates on your progress, eat a health diet, communicate with your healthcare team and practice relaxation techniques. Discussing your care, fears, and triumphs with your healthcare team gives you an opportunity to become secure, comfortable and reassured in your treatment options and daily living. Researching and developing your journal can help you feel more in control of your illness and treatments.

Plan your time, plan your care, and learn to relax in your decisions. The first few years of a chronic illness are stressful times and these techniques can help you figure out your next steps, your daily living, and your physical and mental boundaries. Set the expectation for yourself and those around you as soon as you can. Plan your time so that you can still accomplish important activities to help keep your life fulfilling even when you have changed from who you are.

A Bit About Neuropathy

Neuropathy is a collection of disorders that occurs when nerves of the peripheral nervous are injured or damaged. The peripheral nerves are the system outside of the brain and spinal cord. Neuropathy usually causes pain and numbness resulting from injuries, infections, metabolic disorders, or exposure to toxins. One of the most common causes of neuropathy is diabetes.

There are approximately 150 known types of neuropathy and the causes of all of them are not yet known. Healthcare professionals had a long-standing belief that neuropathy pain is just a symptom of an illness and therefore not a disease. We now know that chronic pain is a disease in itself, and the medical community and public are beginning to look at it in this way. Lack of proof is not evidence that there is no connection; it only means that we need to look harder and do a lot more research!

We are challenged to increase the knowledge of neuropathy conditions. Thirty percent of cases are caused by diabetes, thirty percent are idiopathic, or of an unknown cause, and the other 40% are attributed to autoimmune disorders, tumors, genetic, infections, environmental toxins, and nutritional imbalances. A great source for patients is Dr. Norman Latov's book *Peripheral Neuropathy: When the Numbness, Weakness, and Pain Won't Stop*. This book helps us understand the causes of neuropathies in greater detail. We need to increase awareness, conduct research that is more effective, provide better clinical training for our healthcare professionals, and better tools for diagnosing and treating neuropathy conditions.

It is important that we increase our knowledge as patients and caregivers. Better communication allows for better care and better answers until research catches up to our reality. Too often our healthcare professionals stop short of proper diagnostic procedures due to assumptions, poor attitudes, and limited treatment options available to them. They also get pressure from insurance companies, restrictions on payments for testing and a failure to understand the potential serious impact of these conditions going undiagnosed and undertreated.

Addressing the motor, autonomic, and sensory symptoms can help reduce the impact of the neuropathy. This prevents serious disabilities from developing or developing more rapidly. Research must be done to better the treatment options and develop preventative techniques to lessen the devastating effects of neuropathy.

Webster defines a disease as "a particular destructive process in an organism". A medical dictionary defines a disease as "any deviation from, or interruption of, the normal structure or function of any body part, organ, or system that is manifested by a characteristic set of symptoms and signs and whose etiology, pathology, and prognosis may be known or unknown." With this definition of the word, neuropathy is a disease. Unfortunately, the medical research and the clinical approach to the patient is that neuropathy is NOT seen as a single disease, but as a clinical entity.

Funding for neuropathy research is difficult to obtain because clinical professionals do not fully understand all of the complexities of neuropathy. Far too often, if a patient does not have a known neuropathy condition, healthcare professionals often times say they could not possibly have a neuropathy. Neuropathy is not just a symptom of another disease it can be a disease in itself. When our medical professionals fail to recognize the disease or causes of neuropathy it leads to misdiagnosis, failure to diagnose, and failure of proper treatment. This can cause further damage to the patient. The "do no harm" motto no longer applies when healthcare professionals are working actively on patients but are not up to date on current information. They are blocking progress and possible better outcomes for their patients.

There has to be a better communication between researchers, healthcare professionals, and patients. Far too many people in and out of the medical system have a preconceived notion of what neuropathy is and is not. Medical science has only recently progressed beyond the well-known diseases such as aids, alcoholism, and diabetes. Dr. Bruce Carruthers, MD, CM, FRCP, principal author of *'Fibromyalgia Syndrome: Canadian Clinical Working Group Case Definition, Diagnostic and Treatment Protocols*, notes the clinical approach is important to research in his article *The Importance of Clinical Definitions for Defining and Studying Syndromes*. "A syndrome involves determining the symptoms and how they interact, and how a cluster of symptoms interacts as a group. The establishment of this interaction is essential in clinical practice (and in research)."[4][5]

Healthcare professionals far too often fail to diagnose or treat neuropathy conditions for various reasons. How can we be sure to get to the correct doctor and get the needed treatment for our condition without further delay?

Know your body. Know that neuropathy is not only in the feet but can be in other parts of the

---

[4] Carruthers B, Jain A, et al. "Myalgic Encephalomyelitis/ Chronic Fatigue Syndrome: Clinical Working Case Definition, Diagnostic and Treatment Protocols" *J Chronic Fatigue Syndrome*, 2003, 11: 7-115

[5] Jain A, Carruthers B, et al, "Fibromyalgia Syndrome: Clinical Case Definition, Diagnostic and Treatment Protocols-A Consensus Document" J Musculoskeletal Pain, 2003, 11: 3-107

body. I have had some doctors tell me that neuropathy does not affect the upper body, hands or face, so I could not possibly have neuropathy in my upper body and it must be something else going on.

Know your limitations and your healthcare providers' (HCP) limitations. Sometimes it is difficult for the HCP to understand all of our symptoms or the daily problems we face. There are times when the doctor might believe that you can do something that you know will increase your symptoms or set off a flare. Communicate these limitations to your doctor and find out their knowledge of your condition.

Knowledge is power! Seek credible information, keep your mind open to new treatment options, and provide copies of your research to your treating HCP when necessary. Remember – our providers see many patients day after day and do not always have the time to do the research on new information or upcoming tools. You may be the first one to bring new information to them. This is ok, as long as they are open to learning, communicating, and growing through the process with you.

Through better treatment options, we will be less frustrated as patients and caregivers and can make greater progress in our goal to have better activities of daily living. We also need to encourage our researchers to develop better tools for our treating doctors.

Use a multidisciplinary approach to treatment. Include in your team of providers doctors who specialize in pain management (usually anesthesiologists), internal medicine specialists, neuromuscular neurologists, physical therapists, and psychologists/psychiatrists. Depending on the type of neuropathy you have, you may want to add doctors of immunology, radiology, oncology, hematology (liver), cardiology, pulmonology, orthopedics, urology, gastroenterology, podiatry, as well as other medical disciplines.

When you read books by other patients, or hear of possible new choices in your social circles, be sure to have your own treating HCP consult on these ideas. Patients are not a one size fits all; you may have limitations to a particular modality due to specifics within your own body.

Work with a healthcare provider who works with neuropathy patients on a regular basis. They tend to be more familiar with the daily challenges we face as patients. Until research provides more answers and tools for diagnosing neuropathy, good doctor - patient communication and support from other patients is the solutions of failure to diagnose and treat patients in a timely manner.

Types of Nerves

- Autonomic Nerves - These nerves regulate biological activities that people do not control consciously. (breathing, digesting food, heart)
- Motor Nerves – These nerves control movements of all muscles under conscious control. (e.g. walking, grasping things, talking)
- Sensory nerves – These nerves transmit information about sensory experiences. (feeling a light touch, the pain resulting from a cut)

Some neuropathy affects all three types of nerves, others primarily affect one or two types. In describing a patient's condition, doctors may use terms such as:

- Predominately motor neuropathy
- Predominately sensory neuropathy
- Sensory-motor neuropathy
- Autonomic neuropathy

Identifying Symptoms

Our nervous system is a vast communication network that transmits information to and from the brain/spinal cord to every other part of the body. These messages tell us about our environment and how we are doing physically; how cold we are, to flee from a dangerous situation, burning our hand, balance and coordination. Damage to our nervous system interferes with vital communications. Think of it like the internet. You lose signal strength if something distorts or blocks the signal. Neuropathy sometimes distorts the messages between our body and mind. Our nervous system is bodywide. Each nerve has a highly specialized function coordinating to specific parts of the body so symptoms may vary between patients.

Symptoms can be related to the type of nerves affected. Symptoms can be fluid in nature, meaning that they fluctuate over time. The patient may have days, weeks or years with flaring symptoms. Not all symptoms are experienced by every patient or every neuropathy condition.

Some Symptoms of Neuropathy Conditions

- Bone degeneration
- Breathing difficulty
- Burning pain
- Changes in the skin, hair, and nails
- GI system dysfunction
- Abnormal sexual function
- Blood pressure and vascular constriction issues
- Muscle loss, weakness, wasting
- Nerve pain (neuralgias)
- Organ or gland dysfunction
- Painful cramps and uncontrolled muscle twitching
- Paralysis
- Pricking sensations (paresthesia)
- Organ dysfunction

- Sensitivity to touch
- Increase in sweating
- Numbness / tingling / pins and needles
- Loss of bladder control

Types of Neuropathy

Over 150 types of neuropathy have been identified. Each condition has its own set of symptoms, development, and outcomes. The level of disability and symptoms depends on the type of nerves that are damaged (motor, sensory, or autonomic).

- Acute neuropathy/ acute inflammatory demyelinating neuropathy - symptoms appear suddenly, progress rapidly and resolve slowly as damaged nerves heal, (e.g. Guillain-Barré Syndrome)
- Chronic neuropathy involves symptoms begin subtly and progress slowly. Some people may have periods of relief followed by relapse. Others may reach a plateau stage where symptoms stay the same for many months or years. Some chronic neuropathies worsen over time, but very few types prove fatal unless

complicated by other diseases. Chronic neuropathy can be a symptom of another disorder

- Mononeuritis multiplex - two or more isolated nerves in separate areas of the body are affected
- Mononeuropathy - involves damage to only one nerve
- Polyneuropathy - multiple nerves affecting all limbs are affected (more common)

Acquired Peripheral Neuropathies are Grouped into Three Broad Categories
- Those caused by systemic disease
- Those caused by trauma from external agents
- Those caused by infections or autoimmune disorders affecting nerve tissue

Causes of Neuropathy include
- Physical injury (trauma) to a nerve
- Tumors
- Toxins
- Autoimmune responses

- Nutritional deficiencies
- Alcoholism
- Vascular and metabolic disorders

Most Common Neuropathy Diseases
- Autoimmune Neuropathy
- Autonomic Neuropathy
- Burning Mouth Syndrome
- Carpal Tunnel Syndrome
- Causalgia
- Charcot-Marie-Tooth Disease
- Complex Regional Pain Syndrome / CRPS
- Diabetic Neuropathy
- Fabry Disease
- Fibromyalgia
- Guillain Barre Syndrome
- HIV/AIDS
- Leprosy
- Lupus
- Lyme Disease
- Mediated Pain
- MonoNeuropathy
- Multiple Sclerosis

- Neuralgia
- Neuralgia Post-Infectious
- Neuro Inflammatory Disease
- Peripheral Neuropathy
- Polyneuropathy
- Post-Chemo Neuropathy
- Post-Herpetic
- Post-Surgical Pain
- Reflex Sympathetic Dystrophy/ RSD
- Shoulder Hand Syndrome
- Sympathetically Independent Pain
  Sympathetically
- Toxic Neuropathy
- Trigeminal Neuralgia
- Vasculitic Neuropathy

3

IT PAYS TO ORGANIZE YOUR
HEALTHCARE

One of the best things I did was to get my doctors to communicate with each other. I asked my pain doctor which primary doctor he would recommend, and then asked my primary, which Neurologist, GI, Heart, Lung doctors to use. Then my doctors began to meet on their "common patients" and my team was formed. It was decided that only my primary doctor would order medications and if the other doctors wanted me to try a specific medication or change something, it went through my primary care doctor. This helps when doctors are worried about you being a drug seeker. If only one doctor is prescribing and all of your doctors are in communication, it is less likely that you are drug seeking or an addict.

This is a great benefit for me and it is rare. Therefore, you may need to coordinate with your primary care doctor to make a similar set up happen. The more organized you are, the better your care and the greater success in your outcome. Always order your records and make sure a copy of any healthcare provider is also provided to your primary doctor. You may have to make copies yourself to bring to your primary doctor but it is worth it.

You must take responsibility for your care! Do not leave everything to your doctor. Your providers are your partners in care, but you have the ultimate responsibility. The person who cares about your health and wellbeing the most should be you. So, what can you do to make sure that the right steps are being taken? Listen to your body and track your changes in a daily journal.

- Be sure to track all of your symptoms
  - If you have heart failure track weight changes
  - If you have heart has rhythm problems track your pulse
  - If you have hypertension track your blood pressure
  - If you have pain track your levels and flairs
  - Track when you take you medications and dosages

This kind of home monitoring lets you spot potentially harmful changes before they blossom into real trouble.

- Build a team
- Doctors don't have all the answers
- Seek out the real experts in the areas you need. For instance, a nurse might be a better resource for helping you stop smoking or start exercising and you will get the best nutrition information from a dietitian than a doctor

Treatment Options

As of now, there is no cure for neuropathy; however, there are many therapies and treatment options. You must research and figure out what is best for you and your specific neuropathy condition. It is important to have any underlying condition treated as soon as possible, followed up by symptomatic treatment. By taking care of your underlying condition and your symptoms, it can prevent new damage. Having injuries treated in a timely manner can help prevent permanent damage.

Your options start with things you can do on your own to reduce physical and emotional effects such as:

- Approved physical therapy: active and passive forms of exercise can reduce cramps and prevent muscle wasting in paralyzed limbs
- Avoid toxin exposure (pesticides, additives)
- Correcting vitamin deficiencies
- Diet and nutrition: use dietary strategies to improve GI symptoms (balanced diet, health food)

- Following a physician-supervised physical therapy program
- Limiting or avoiding alcohol consumption
- Maintaining an optimal weight
- Proper wound care (especially in diabetes)
- Stop smoking: smoking constricts blood vessels that supply nutrients to the peripheral nerves and can worsen neuropathic symptoms

Nerve pain is often difficult to get under control. Multiple options are available and can help mild to severe pain. Find the options that help control your pain the best. Some of those may include assistive devices, medical procedures, or over-the-counter/prescription medications. Below are some options from which to choose. Be sure to consult your healthcare professional team as to what would be best for you.

Goal Creation and Treatment Plans Should Include:
- Drug management
- Family/ social adjustment

- Improve the patient's quality of life and psycho-social functioning
- Increasing mobilization/ range of motion through physical therapy to help prevent progression and worsening of symptoms
- Keep a daily journal
- Medical team coordination

Milestones are Considered Successful Treatments by Many Neuropathy Patients:

- Ability to perform physical therapy with marked improvement in muscle strength
- Able to achieve a full night's sleep repeatedly
- Decreased need for narcotics
- Diminished depression
- Improved thinking
- Increase in daily chores and activities
- Increase in stamina
- Lower pain levels, or pain controlled with low to moderate consideration
- Diminished swelling of the affected arm or leg

Medications

When taking medications it is a good idea to consult with your pharmacist about any interactions with other medications you are taking, possible side effects, and correct dosage. Many times medications are prescribed that interact with other medications. Your doctor may not realize you are not taking a medication or not know of the interaction possibilities. For example, I thought if the doctor kept writing a script for a medication it was safe to keep taking. Turns out the NSAIDS are known to cause bleeding ulcers and are meant for short-term use. I did not know that. My doctor knew I had a chronic condition and I refused to take narcotics, so I took what he offered. I ended up in the hospital with bleeding ulcers.

It is important to know the risks of that medication and to do your own research. Do not rely only on your doctor. This is important to discuss with a pharmacist. Ask about the maximum time a person should be on the medication. Find out what time of day to take the medication and if it should be taken on an empty stomach.

Below are some of the medications often prescribed to patients with a neuropathy condition.

- Anti-Seizure: Carbamazepine (Tegretol), Gabapentin (Neurontin), Phenytoin (Dilantin)
- Antidepressants: Amitriptyline, Nortriptyiline, Antidepressants for pain control and treating psychological effects related to prolonged pain
- Aspirin and acetaminophen also known as Tylenol
- Corticoid steroids - to reduce inflammation and swelling. Example: Calcitonin spray
- If no lasting relief is achieved after six weeks a stronger longer-lasting narcotic for breakthrough pain as well as antidepressants are usually prescribed
- Intrathecal drug delivery - drugs delivered into the spinal fluid through the spinal cord or delivered through a pain pump. Pain pump drugs include Morphine, Baclofen, and Clonidine. Baclofen is often successful for severe Dystonia as well
- Ketamine or Lidocaine infusions are effective for approximately 80% of patients

- Medications may offer enough pain relief to begin physical therapy exercises
- Muscle relaxants: Baclofen (Lioresal), Klonopin
- Non-steroidal anti-inflammatory drugs (N-SAIDS) or Ibuprofen
- Adhesive patches - usually reserved for severe, chronic pain. These include Lidocaine, and Fentanyl
- Opioid - used for widespread pain, Morphine, Nucynta (Tapentadol), Opana (Oxymorphone), Ultram (Tramadol)

Infusion Therapy

Infusion therapy can be done with Ketamine, Lidocaine, Metamine, IVIg, Naltrexone, and even stem cells. Below is some additional information for Ketamine infusions and IVIg infusions, but you must consult with your doctor as to what is best for you. Patients may be excluded from a particular treatment option because of different reasons. Top-rated United States-based Neurological doctors have said that Ketamine infusion therapy is perhaps the best treatment for RSD and other Neurological conditions.

There are three forms of Ketamine protocols that are administered through intravenous means. Those are coma, outpatient, and inpatient. All three protocols have opponents and proponents in the medical field, but for many RSD patients this option has become a glimmer of hope and possibility of returning us to a life of normalcy. Dr. Robert J. Schwartzman, a leading specialist in RSD and Ketamine protocols says this is the closest treatment to a cure and he sees a day where the Ketamine protocols become the leading treatment for RSD patients. Per the National Institute on Drug Abuse Research Report Series: *Hallucinogens and Dissociative Drugs*, 2001 – Ketamine is an odorless, tasteless drug that is found in liquid, pill, and powder form. Ketamine is classified as a type of dissociative drug. It alters the actions of the neurotransmitter glutamate throughout the brain. Glutamate is involved in perception of pain, response to the environment, and memory.

Outpatient Protocol: The outpatient version is usually done over a 5 to 10 day period. Some doctors do a few days, weeks or spread it out over a few months. Each infusion last approximately four hours. After a patient receives inpatient or coma Ketamine treatments, they are typically given outpatient infusions as "boosters" over the next few months to a year or so to enhance the lasting effects of the pain lowering benefits. Of course, doctors will have their own protocol and we are just listing a typical version. This version was approved by the FDA in 2002 and is currently used by doctors across the country.

A recent outpatient IV Ketamine study for the treatment of CRPS/RSD study was done by Drexel University College of Medicine doctors and healthcare professionals demonstrated a statistically significant reduction in many pain parameters ($p < 0.05$). The report was featured in a journal publication called *PAIN*. This is a landmark study as it is the first study utilizing an active placebo as a control. Professionals involved are Robert J. Schwartzman, MD; Guillermo M. Alexander, Ph.D.; John R. Grothusen, Ph.D.; Terry

Paylor RN; Erin Reichenberger MS; and Marielle Perreault BS.

In Patient Protocol: This treatment is typically done over 5 to 7 continuous days of IV infusion with a combination of Ketamine and Clonidine while the patient is in the hospital. The patient will typically undergo outpatient booster treatments after the inpatient protocol is complete. This protocol is being done by doctors and hospitals since 2002 in more than five states. Hundreds of patients have done this procedure with a high success rate. Although all patients are different, outcomes are continually improving and the success rate is increasing as well. A successful case is considered remission.

Coma Protocol: Patients are placed into an induced coma with a high dose of Ketamine, for 5 to 7 days. Patients travel to Mexico or Germany with a team of American doctors as this procedure is not yet approved by the FDA. It will be difficult to get approval because the FDA is requiring a double blind study. A double-blind study is an experimental procedure in which neither the subjects of the experiment nor the persons administering the experiment know the critical aspects of the experiment. This type of study is used to guard against both experimenter bias and placebo effects. Due to the complications that may arise when putting someone into a coma, any type of double-blind study of this nature is going to be very difficult. There are a number of patients who remain in remission after years have passed from this type of infusion.

IVIG is given as a plasma protein replacement therapy (IgG) for immune deficient patients who have decreased or abolished antibody production capabilities. In these immune deficient patients, IVIG is administered to maintain adequate antibodies, levels to prevent infections, and resistance to passive immunity. Treatment is given every 3 to 4 weeks. In the case of patients with autoimmune disease, IVIG is administered at a high dose (generally 1-2 grams IVIG per kg body weight) to attempt to decrease the severity of the autoimmune diseases such as Dermatomyositis.

A use of IVIG for a neurological disease is typically dispensed at 2 grams per kilogram of body weight and is implemented for three to six months over a five-day period once a month. Then maintenance therapy of 100 to 400 mg/kg of body weight every 3 to 4 weeks follows. Routine use of IVIG is common practice, sometimes long-term, and is considered safe.

Complications of IVIG therapy include:
- Acute renal (kidney) failure
- Venous thrombosis
- Aseptic meningitis
- Allergic/anaphylactic reactions; for example, anaphylactic shock, especially in iga deficient patients, who by definition can still produce igg antibodies (iga deficient patients are more likely to produce igg against the IVIg administration than normal patients)
- Damage such as hepatitis caused directly by antibodies contained in the pooled IVIg
- Dermatitis (peeling of the skin of the palms and soles)
- Severe headache
- Infection (such as HIV or viral hepatitis) by contaminated blood product
- Pulmonary edema from fluid overload

Physical Therapy

Physical therapy and medications are commonly used as harmonizing therapies in the beginning of treatment. If there is no relief from the physical therapy in one to two months then Sympathetic Nerve Blocks (SNB) are typically considered. The SNB's are done in conjunction with drug therapy. Physical therapy for neuropathy patients who are still in severe pain should include traction, stretching and massage, and no to low weights. Therapy should be done to alleviate or lower pain levels, restore function to the limb, reduce swelling, reduce stiff joints, and strengthen your muscles. Make sure to find a physical therapist that specializes in chronic pain and neuropathy conditions specifically, if possible. If it does not feel right, speak up and do not do it. Have open communication with your physical therapist so you get the greatest benefits.

On your good days, try a few new things in your environment and physical activity. This can increase function, range of motion, increase your muscle strength and improve balance and posture.

Do what you can do at your level. It will be different for all of us. Moving will increase your health, function of your affected limbs, and help with constipation and gastrointestinal issues caused by the neuropathy conditions and medications. Movement increases your blood circulation that helps with atrophy and can decrease hypersensitivity.

Using a combined therapy approach may lead you to faster relief. The other therapy methods sometimes incorporated include biofeedback, hot compresses, elevation, light massage, range of motion exercises, mirror box therapy, and hydrotherapy. Patients can combine counseling, physical therapy and a drug regimen for better relief. Doing this can help us stay on track with our treatment plan and increase the benefits of physical therapy.

Questions to ask when consulting with a physical therapist:
- What is your understanding of neuropathy
- When do you feel weight bearing exercises are appropriate

- If I become nauseous after stretching, should I continue with the stretching
- Do you believe pain is no gain
- Do you believe neuropathy patients should use ice to lower inflammation

Non-invasive/Less-invasive procedures

Typically, non or less invasive procedures should be done first. These include sympathetic nerve blocks, tens unit, radiofrequency ablations, patches, and hyperbaric oxygen therapy.

Sympathetic Nerve Blocks

Sympathetic nerve blocks (SNB) do not block motor activity so you can remain mobile and active, which offers you a better range of motion. Your range of motion and exercises can increase during the time the nerve block has reduced the degree of pain.

Tens Unit

The tens unit provides electrical nerve stimulation in small amounts to the nerves to overcome the sensation of pain. It is a trick to your nerves. Think about when you have hurt yourself on something in the past. Your reaction is to rub the area. This causes a good sensation to be sent the brain, which can sometimes help forget the pain. The tens unit are portable and available for self-treatment with a small unit. Negative effects can include skin rashes from the sticky side of the electrode. People with pacemakers and pregnant women should not use the tens unit.

Topical Pain Patches

Topical pain patches such as Lidoderm, Fentanyl, and Clonidine as well as lotions can be easily applied. Be sure to check with your doctor about potential side effects.

Acupuncture

Acupuncture is an alternative medicine methodology. It treats patients by inserting thin solid needles into acupuncture points in the skin. Stimulating these points can correct imbalances in the flow of Qi through channels known as meridians. Acupressure is often thought of as acupuncture without the needles and is less invasive.

Hyperbaric Oxygen Therapy

Hyperbaric oxygen therapy advances wound healing, increases the delivery of oxygen to injured tissues, encourages greater blood vessel formation, and preserves damaged tissues. In the chamber, you may feel pressure in the ears similar to the sensation felt when landing in an airplane. The chamber may become slightly warmer during the first few minutes of treatment and will be cooler during the last few minutes. In some multi-person chambers, patients can watch television, a movie; listen to the radio or just rest.

Radiofrequency Ablations

Radiofrequency Ablations (RFA) is a medical procedure sometimes used to treat severe chronic pain, where radiofrequency waves are used to produce heat. This heat is targeted on specifically identified nerves. By generating heat around the nerve, its ability to transmit pain signals to the brain is destroyed, thus ablating the nerve. The nerves to be ablated are identified through injections through local anesthesia, such as lidocaine, prior to the RFA procedure. If the local anesthesia injections provide temporary pain relief, then RFA is performed on the nerves that responded well to the injections. The RFA procedure has risks such as new nerve injuries, bleeding, allergic reactions to the medications being used, seizures, and the stress and fear about the procedure. I underwent over 35 of these procedures at a pulsed level verses regular level. It is important that you have a competent pain management specialist because of the variety of complications can be involved in performing the procedure. My suggestion is if you choose to receive an RFA, only get this procedure from a trained professional who has performed this procedure on a regular basis. It is important to notify your doctor of any side effects you may have or complications noted after the procedure. The major drawback of this procedure is that nerves regenerate overtime.

Orthopedic surgery/ Invasive surgery

The more invasive a procedure is the harder it can be on your body. Depending on your doctors expertise they may only offer a more invasive procedure. Please do your research and understand what the benefits and drawbacks are of each procedure. Three of the most invasive are sympathectomy, spinal cord or brain stimulator, and pain pump placement.

Sympathectomy

Sympathectomy is a procedure that has high risks and the outcome varies from patient to patient this should be used as a last resort. Carefully weigh the risks of the procedure and communicate with your doctor in great detail. Once the nerve bundle is removed, there is nothing for the doctor to treat if the pain returns. Sympathectomy involves cutting out the sympathetic ganglion nerve bundle which is located in a specific area along the spinal cord. If it is determined that the source of the neuropathy pain is sympathetically maintained (SMP), in which pain is reduced with a sympathetic nerve block than this may be an option. However if the pain is determined to be sympathetically independent pain (SIP) a sympathectomy is not a procedure that will benefit you. Once removed it is permanent. Even if you have SMP, it may turn into SIP down the road with an additional insult to the body, so the risks are high for failure from this procedure. If you have chosen to receive a full sympathectomy, you will be limited or out of treatment options if it fails. With the possible risks, make sure that you are an appropriate candidate for this procedure and that you are willing to undergo the procedure in spite of the risks. This procedure does not always work even when SMP is involved.

Spinal Cord/Brain Stimulator

Spinal cord neuromodulation complications such as infections and the spread of neuropathy symptoms to other parts of your body are at a higher risk. The idea with this choice is the spinal cord interrupting the pain signal to the brain. Spinal cord stimulators (SCS) have an effect on the entire central nervous system. Before a SCS is implanted permanently, you should have a period with a temporary stimulator. The surgical implantation is described as feeling like an electrical current, but is reported by patients to be far less bothersome compared to the pain of neuropathy conditions. The spinal stimulator is not a cure but in many cases it can reduce the pain to a more manageable level.

However, only a small number of neuropathy patients who have the stimulator have benefits that last more than two years, and most have complications such as moved leads, infections, quick draining of batteries and feeling of internal shocks in your spine. Any patients undergoing radiation, or have pacemakers, or are exposed to alarm detection devices should not consider this option.

Complications associated with surgical implantation of the SCS include significant bleeding in the epidural space, infection in the epidural space could potentially lead to meningitis or an epidural abscess. Surgical complications associated with SCS include injury to the spinal cord, paralysis, accumulation of fluid in the power source site, and spinal headaches. In addition, tenderness at the generator/receiver (power source) is common until healing occurs, but persistent pain at the stimulator site is possible, as is tissue damage at the site of the stimulator lead and connecting cables.

There are also issues of mechanical complications with the system. These can include dislodgment of the lead, movement of the lead, breaks in the wiring or problems with the power source. Occasionally, loss of pain relief in a painful area can occur even if stimulation is still felt in that area.

Pain Pump

Pain pumps are surgically implanted to deliver pain medication directly to the fluid around the spinal cord, providing pain relief with a small fraction of the medication needed if taken orally. [6] They are also called "intrathecal drug delivery systems." Typically, patients take daily medications orally that are processed through the

---

[6] Brogan SE. Intrathecal therapy for the management of cancer pain. *Curr Pain Headache Rep*. 2006;10:254-259

GI system before making it into the blood stream. With pain pumps, the medication is released directly into the fluid surrounding your spinal cord, which may lead to fewer or tolerable drug side effects. The system has two parts, the pump that is the part of the device, which stores the pain medication and the catheter, which is inserted into your spine. Both are placed under the skin. Instead of taking a daily dose of medication orally, the pump is programmed to release the dosage. When emptied you return to your doctor for a refill.

Although many patients do get relief with the pain pump, it is important to note a few facts. Realistic expectation of the amount of relief expected and mindset of the patient is important going into the procedure. The pain pump does not eliminate the source of your pain or cure any underlying disease, but it can help manage your pain. After multiple studies, it is also known that opioids activate Glia cells which are part of our flight fight system. When Glia cells are activated, the patient experiences pain. With a neuropathy you are experiencing activated Glia. Different types of medications can be used in the pain pump, but when an opioid is used this can excite the Glia further. However, the opioid also is able to work on the brain and affect mood. Although we are in pain, we do not care as much. Some people accept this as pain relief and if this is the choice you make with your doctor it can always be removed surgically if you decide to pursue other options. Keep in mind that the surgery to implant and remove the device is trauma to your body. Some neuropathy conditions can worsen with new trauma such as Reflex Sympathetic Dystrophy (RSD). If a pain pump is an option for you, your doctor will work with you to select the pain treatment system best suited to your needs.

Assistive Devices

A goal for increasing activities of daily living might include the use of assistive devices. I look at them as a way to get more activities done each day. I was unable to walk distances, so I got a scooter and was able to ride two blocks over to our mailbox area to pick up the mail. My husband had to add this to his long list of other things I needed assistance with daily. Once I got my scooter it gave me more freedom to adjust to my disabilities and environment and I was able to accomplish more, relieving duties to my husband/caregiver.

If there is a need, a device can be used to assist that need. Many of them are covered by insurance, while others can be purchased over the counter at pharmacies and durable equipment locations. Devices can help reduce pain and lessen the impact of physical disability.

- Bath lift - Works by electrically lowering and raising the user into and out of the bath tub
- Bathroom stool in the shower can be great if you deal with proprioception (balance) issues or leg pain
- Canes can assist with balance and gait issues
- Grab rails and poles are useful for helping you to get in and out of the bath and also reduce the risk of slipping
- Hand or foot braces can compensate for muscle weakness and alleviate nerve compression
- Help prevent foot injuries in people with a loss of pain sensation (common in diabetes)
- Long handled sponges, foot and toe washers, and hair washers can make a real difference.

- Mechanical ventilation can provide essential life support if breathing becomes severely impaired
- Orthopedic Shoes - Some of the most common foot problems can be treated with specially made shoes
- Transfer benches allow you to easily transfer from a wheelchair or power chair to the bath or shower
- Wheelchairs and electric scooters help with mobility problems in and out of the house

Alternative Treatment

There is a variety of alternative treatments to mainstream medicine and it has never been more popular. Some doctors are even embracing complementary and alternative approaches to treating patients. As our health field progresses and grows with new research alternative treatment options change. The National Center for Complementary and Alternative Medicine (NCCAM), funds scientific research and splits alternative medicine into five categories: whole medical systems; mind-body medicine;

biologically based practices; body-based practices; and energy medicine. The difference in each treatment option is not always clear and some treatments may fall into more than one category.

Some examples include:
- Ancient Healing
- Art Therapies
- Chiropractic
- Calmare Therapy
- Dietary Supplements (Selenium, Glucosamine Sulfate and SAME)
- Herbs (Ginseng, Ginkgo, Marijuana, and Echinacea)
- Homeopathy
- Magnet Therapy
- Massage
- Meditation/Prayer
- Mirror Box Therapy
- Music Therapy
- Naturopathy
- Oils / Lotions
- Osteopathic Manipulation

- Prayer
- Qi Gong or Reiki Exercises
- Relaxation Techniques
- Therapeutic Touch

Many mainstream providers do not receive class training on alternative treatment options so they do not feel comfortable addressing this area or they do not believe in it. Some providers need to see scientific research documentation before they will even consider the option. Since they do not get this in their mainstream classes they are not getting the research documents on the options. As provider education on these treatment options grows, we are seeing an increase in their openness to considering the treatments as viable choices for their patients.

It is important to have the research and testing at standards used in mainstream medicine. Options given to patients need to be safe and effective. Some scientific evidence does exist for alternative treatments, but not enough and some key questions still need to be answered. Finding funds for this research tends to be a major obstacle as there is not the medical industry backing. It is troublesome that many practitioners of alternative medicine may exaggerate the outcome or use the data of the people who did benefit from it and leaving out the ones who do not. This makes it seem to be a cure or have a higher percentage of helping when it does not.

You should keep your mainstream provider in the loop on any alternative treatment options you do plan to try. There can be associated risks and it is important to speak with a medical professional about what they may be. This is to help you understand if the benefits outweigh the risks and any possible medication interactions that may occur. This is an especially good idea if you are pregnant, have a chronic care condition, or take prescription medications.

One alternative option that has been in the news a lot lately is medical marijuana. Medical marijuana falls into the Naturopathy category. Although I have not yet tried this option, I have done a lot of research on it. After researching, I believe medical marijuana can help these conditions, but due to the different growing methods and non-standardization of the industry, it is hard to get verifiable detailed study on all of the benefits.

This is not an exhaustive list of the conditions that may be helped by using cannabis.

- AIDS: (acquired immune deficiency syndrome) is the final stage of HIV disease, which causes severe damage to the immune system
- Anorexia: an eating disorder characterized by refusal to maintain a healthy body weight
- Anxiety: a feeling of apprehension or fear, the source of which is not always known or recognized
- Arthritis: inflammation of one or more joints, which results in pain, swelling, stiffness, and limited movement
- Autism: autistic spectrum disorders are a group of developmental disabilities that can cause significant social, communication and behavioral challenges
- Breast Cancer: cannabis study suggesting that a particular compound may be effective at taming metastasizing breast cancer cells with low toxicity

- Cachexia: physical wasting with loss of weight and muscle mass caused by disease
- Cancer: a group of diseases characterized by uncontrolled cell division leading to growth of abnormal tissue
- Crohn's Disease: an inflammatory bowel disease (IBD), causing inflammation of the digestive tract lining This can lead to abdominal pain, severe diarrhea and malnutrition
- Depression: a common condition that presents with depressed mood, loss of interest or pleasure, feelings of guilt or low self-worth, disturbed sleep or appetite, low energy, and poor concentration
- Epilepsy: a disorder that results from the surges in electrical signals inside the brain, causing recurring seizures
- Fibromyalgia: a constellation of symptoms that include widespread aching, stiffness, fatigue, and the presence of specific body tender points
- Glaucoma: a group of eye diseases characterized by damage to the optic nerve

usually caused by raised pressure (IOP) within the eye

- Insomnia: chronic inability to fall asleep or to enjoy uninterrupted sleep
- Irritable bowel syndrome (IBS): Anecdotal evidence suggests that use of cannabis reduces associated symptoms
- Mesothelioma: at least one study looking at cannabis for chemotherapy patients (Harvard University) that showed THC, the active ingredient in cannabis, slashed tumor growth in common lung cancer by 50% and also reduced the spread of the cancer
- Migraine: a severe recurring headache, usually affecting only one side of the head, characterized by sharp pain and often accompanied by nausea, vomiting, and visual disturbances
- Multiple Sclerosis: a chronic autoimmune disorder affecting movement, sensation, and bodily functions Caused by destruction of the myelin insulation covering nerve fibers in the brain and spinal cord

- Nausea: a feeling of sickness in the stomach characterized by an urge to vomit
- Pain: an unpleasant sensation occurring in varying degrees of severity. Can be a consequence of injury or disease
- PTSD: (post traumatic stress disorder) a mental health condition triggered by a terrifying event. Symptoms may include flashbacks, nightmares, severe anxiety, uncontrollable thoughts about the event
- Rheumatoid Arthritis: It's been known, anecdotally at least, for many years that cannabis can help ease the painful symptoms of rheumatoid arthritis

States where Medical Marijuana is Legal

The states below have passed medical marijuana laws. Other states currently have legislation pending. As of yet, there are still Federal laws prohibiting the use of marijuana. Other forms such as Marinol and THC pills are available in even more states.

Alaska	Colorado
Arizona	Delaware
California	Hawaii

Maine	New Mexico
Michigan	Oregon
Montana	Rhode Island
Nevada	Vermont
New Jersey	Washington

Requesting Healthcare Records

When it comes to healthcare records there are laws to ensure the patients confidentially. The federal government passed what we now know as HIPAA laws. HIPAA stands for the Health Insurance Portability and Accountability Act of 1996. Most healthcare providers now have an authorization form for use or disclosure of your protected information. You simply have to complete the form and sign it, then submit it to the provider or hospital for your records. This will allow the providers to speak with whomever you dictate on your forms about your care.

The HIPAA laws also provide some protection for employees and their families when they change their health insurance coverage. The law now prohibits health insurance plans from denying coverage based on poor health. It also guarantees health insurance renewal, in most cases, regardless of current health conditions and the right to purchase coverage.

One thing I have learned is how important it is to keep a copy of all of your medical records. My insurance companies have tried to force me into "step therapy" and without my medical records it would have been very difficult and long process to get through. I save my providers time as well, when I can fill out the insurance forms for appeals and send them over for the doctor to just review and forward on. Just this year I was again faced with a step therapy request. The insurance company said, "If you have already tried the other medications with fail, your doctor should have done the Medform 3500, which is completed and sent into a clearing house." There is voluntary reporting form 3500, and the 3500A that is for issues that are mandatory to report. I went online and found the form and directions on the FDA government website. [7] Once I filled in all of the information, I copied it, attached the pertinent records, and sent it to my doctor. He finished

---

[7] www.fda.gov/Safety/MedWatch/HowToReport

completing it (using the records I attached) and signed and faxed it in. Within a week, my medication was covered and they dropped the step therapy requirement.

Your medical record is comprised of all information generated during your treatment with all healthcare providers. The providers keep track of many aspects of your treatment, including personal, financial, social, and medical information. Many providers are using written forms and notes, but over the past few years, there are great electronic medical record keeping programs that are coming to the market. I am seeing more and more the providers coming in with their laptop and all of my information is in my electronic file. It is important to know what is in your record.

After you order and receive your copies, go through them and check for errors. Check everything because these records are used as a means of communication between your healthcare professionals, hospital staff, physical therapist, etc. They are a legal documentation of the care you have received, a verification of services and many insurance companies request them in chronic care cases to decide on approval of treatment options. The records also serve as basic data for research and education purposes.

You can typically obtain your medical records by writing out a request or filling out a premade form from the provider.

Your record request should include the following: [8]

- Date of the request
- Full Name
- Date of birth
- Social security number
- Telephone number
- Name, address, fax, and telephone number where the records are to be sent
- Purpose of the request (typically, there can be a charge for ordering your records). Each state has different laws on how much can be charged, for instance, there is a law in Arizona that if the records are being used for continuing care, the provider cannot charge you

[8] Sample in The Pain Code Journal

- Specific items or dates of service needed
- Any restrictions on the request
- Date this authorization expires (authorizations must be less than one year old)
- A statement in writing indicating that the patient knows that they have a right to revoke this authorization at any time
- A statement indicating that the patient knows that signing this authorization is not a condition of obtaining treatment
- A statement indicating that the patient understands the potential for the protected health information to be re-disclosed by the recipient and no longer protected
- The signature of the patient or, if the patient is a child, the parent or guardian. If signed by a personal representative, a description of his/her authority to act for the individual and a copy of the document giving that authority. Records are not usually released while a patient is still hospitalized because they are incomplete

If you are in a state that is able to charge for copies of your medical records, you may save some money asking for specific documents or all recent major reports rather than requesting the entire record. Most of my requests have been filled with in 5 to 10 days but it may take up to one month. If you have not heard back in 30 business days, you may want to call or send a written follow up request. A few providers are offering your records online and others may provide it to you in electronic form if you provide them a flash drive.

Check with each provider as to the method they prefer. Some providers will fax medical records and some will only fax them to another healthcare provider in cases of immediate emergency. Your records are the physical property of the provider, however, the patient controls the release of the information contained in their record. In addition, if you are moving away from your provider, you may request your entire file so that you may provide it to the next provider who will be taking over your care. Providers must keep a copy of your records for a particular amount of years. In some states it is seven, others it is ten years, although most providers keep them longer.

There are instances where your records can be shared without your consent. Such as in response to a subpoena or court order, to certain government agencies, to someone who holds your power of attorney, to someone you have designated as your healthcare surrogate, to another healthcare providers, for continued care, and to your healthcare insurer to obtain reimbursement for your care. Otherwise, you must give permission for anyone other than a member of your healthcare team to have access to your records.

In some cases where the parent is still claiming their child as a dependent but the child is 18 or older the parent, although responsible for the bills, would not have permission to view the records unless written permission from the patient is given. For children under 18, only the parent or court appointed guardian may authorize release of the patient's medical information. In cases of divorce, both parents have rights to the medical records unless a court has severed the parental rights of one or both of the parents. If a person passes away, only the next of kin or representative of the estate may request medical records.

Medication Management

When it comes to managing medication the more you know about your condition the better equipped you will be to understand which medication to take, the side effects to watch for and when to take it. It is also a great idea for your caregiver to know. There are many times when I am not doing well where and my husband says, "you are dizzy, have you taken XX yet? When was the last time you took it?" or "We are going to go out later to get groceries, so take your pill now so you won't be asleep when we go and you will be more comfortable." Having someone help me with this is great because sometimes I feel so awful that I cannot remember to even take the medication or what I have taken. The Pain Code Journal has a place to list your medications and information.

I have a pill container because remembering to take your pills everyday can be tough. I have overdosed a few times because I forgot I already took my medication. So I now have a pill box that is a two week supply separated morning and night pills. It is also important to take the pills at the same time each day, especially when pills are time released versions. This helps to keep the level of medication consistent in your body.

It is important to know why you are taking each medication, how best to take them (before/after eating), and any side effects that you may experience. Find out what your doctor wants you to do for each medication and verify it with your pharmacist. Be sure to never break or split time-release pills. Breaking the seal can be very dangerous as your body can receive the dose of the whole pill too quickly and it can become deadly.

You should also carry a list of your medications and doses at all times in your purse or wallet. Do not drive under the influence of medication that affects your cognitive thinking. It is also a good idea not to drive while taking medication causing drowsiness or when you are distracted by pain. If you are taking a medication and it is making you sick or causing side effects that you cannot tolerate, talk to your physician about adjusting the dose or changing the medication. If side effects include trouble breathing, rash, or other more severe symptoms head to a local emergency room for immediate assistance. If your doctor tells you to discontinue a medication, dispose of it properly and immediately. It is also a good idea to keep medications without childproof caps away from children.

If you decide you no longer want to continue a medication get your provider's guidance. Some medications can be stopped immediately but many require you to titrate off them. Read the medication bottle label and inserts carefully, they contain important information such as medication name, dosage, prescribing doctor, and expiration dates. This can help you avoid taking a medication too long and having adverse affects from long-term use.

If you are a drinker be sure to discuss with your provider or pharmacist if it is safe to drink with any of the prescriptions or over-the-counter medications you are taking. If you have more than one treating doctor prescribing medications be sure to tell them what you are taking.

When possible have one prescribing doctor to help prevent medication interactions and complications. You should also update your pharmacy records to include all of the medications that you take. This list should also include any over-the-counter medications you take. Finally, as I mentioned before, use a pill organizer, especially when taking several medications a day.

A complete list of Disposal Recommendations can be found at the FDA site. Some basic rules are to dispose of medication once the expiration date has passed. The patient should follow any specific disposal instructions on the drug label or patient information that accompanies the medication.

Some medications such as inhalants have hazardous material disposal requirements. If no instructions are given, you can crush and mix medications with coffee grounds, cat litter, or food scraps. Then seal them in a bag or a container (such as a margarine tub or jar) and discard them in the regular trash. You can always ask your pharmacist if you are not sure how to dispose of your medications. Each year there are "Take Back" events in many communities across the United

States that you can participate in. [9]   Find out more from your local pharmacist or police station.

End of Life Decisions

This is a hard topic but a necessary one for adults. You need to plan for end-of-life even if you are very healthy, but especially when you have a chronic condition. When you are facing a chronic condition that gets progressively worse, the sooner you plan the better off the care can be when it comes time for the last days of your chronic care. Be sure to put your wishes in writing and have it notarized if possible. [8]

You must decide if you want the most aggressive care until the very end, hospice care, or a do-not-resuscitate (DNR) order. Doing this simple step can save you and your loved ones a lot of confusion and anguish when the time comes that a decision needs to be made. Being a planner will make your life simpler. We plan our lives, we plan for our estates after we die, but many skip the process of planning our end-of-life wishes. When

---

[9] FDA Consumer Health Information/U. S. Food and Drug Administration, April 2011, www.fda.gov/downloads/Drugs

we do not at least think about it and tell our caregivers/family members when they must take over, we are vulnerable, and they may not do what gives you the most understanding, comfort, and dignity. Try to confront and understand any fears you might have such as:

- Are your legal and financial affairs in order
- Ask your doctor for guidance in preparing advance directives
- Ask your doctor what you might expect to happen when you begin to feel worse
- Being alone
- Dying in a strange place
- Leaving loved ones
- Loss of dignity
- Not being clearly understood
- Overly-sedated
- Pain not being relieved
- Unfinished projects
- Your loved ones financial resources

If there is someone in your life that you want to know your plan but they are scared to hear it, use conversations "openers".

- Recall a family event
- Share your values and beliefs, your hopes and fears about the end stage of your life and theirs
- Talk about whom you wish to leave a possession to
- Talking about a future event where you might not be present
- Whom you would like to have near if you were seriously ill
- Talk to a religious adviser about spiritual concerns

It is surprising the family members who disagree over what would be done for an ill relative. Planning an advance directive makes your wishes clear and takes the burden off the family in a stressful time. The advance directive is instructions for your providers and family so they know how to care for you or if you wish to refuse treatment.

It is important to complete a written advanced directive for your benefit and your caregivers/ families benefit. Decide whom you want to make decisions for you if you are not able to make your own, on both financial matters and health care decisions. Keep in mind that the same person may not be right for both. Decide on what medical treatments are acceptable to you. You need to make up your mind as to if you wish to be resuscitated if you stop breathing and/or your heart stops? If you are seriously ill or terminally ill, you may want to stay at home, in a hospital or somewhere else that is comfortable for you.

Determine financial issues of being cared for. Do you have adequate health insurance and life insurance benefits? Keep all your insurance papers in a handy location. Give a copy to a trusted relative or friend or let them know where they can find it when needed. Be sure to tell a trusted person(s) where these documents are located. You should also write out instructions for your funeral and how it will be paid for. [10]

It is a good idea to have a durable power of attorney, advanced directives, and living will. The durable power of attorney is for financial affairs, the advance directive and living will are to indicate

---

[10] Family Caregiver Alliance, Where to Find My Important Papers, caregiver.org/caregiver

the instructions for your care. These are legally binding documents that you prepare, or have prepared for you to sign, that designates a trusted person to act for you if you become debilitated. Make sure you have a valid up-to-date will or trust documents if desired or needed. You may want to choose different people for your financial affairs and your healthcare.

These documents are instructions that communicate your wishes and are used when you are unable to speak for yourself. Any healthcare facility that receives Medicare and Medicaid payments is required to provide information to the patients on preparing an advanced directive and the right to refuse treatment. Every state recognizes advanced directives but the laws governing each state vary.

The person you designate as your "agent" will be able to make decisions for you regarding your healthcare, from minor needs (flu shot) to major needs (surgery). They decide if the provider proceeds with life-sustaining procedures. Choose someone who is good under pressure, because many decisions regarding health have to made and changed rapidly. Trust in the person you pick because someone has to make decisions for you when you are too ill.

If you do not make plans the hospital staff and your spouse or child will make the best decision they can, but often times without direction from you ahead of time. You must rely on their ideals and the provider's medical expertise which may go against your beliefs. Keep in mind that most healthcare providers will proceed with good intentions and have been trained to do all they can to keep you alive. The ways all of these people choose to keep you as comfortable as they can may not be what you want. In addition, if you do not name an agent, a court can appoint one to make decisions for you and when a family member cannot be reached or are in disagreement, the judge may appoint a public agent. It would be best to make the plans and decisions ahead of time to ensure your wishes are carried out to the best of the providers and your agent's ability.

Living Will

You can use the sample Living Will form in *The Pain Code Journal* to create a personalized form for decisions now about your medical care if you are ever in a terminal condition, a persistent vegetative state or an irreversible coma. You should talk to your doctor about what these terms mean.

The Living Will states what choices you would have made for yourself if you were able to communicate. It is your written directions to your health care representative if you have one, your family, physician, and any other person who might be in a position to make medical decisions for you. Talk to your family members, friends, and others you trust about your choices. In addition, it is a good idea to talk with professionals such as your doctor, clergyperson and a lawyer before you complete and sign your Living Will. [11]

---

[11] Adapted, Original developed by the Office of the Arizona Attorney General, TERRY GODDARD, www.azag.gov , 2007

4

FACING FINANCIAL CHALLENGES

Being that 1 in 2.66 people in America are dealing with a condition that causes chronic pain at some point in their life, the demand is getting even greater for community resources. There are a wide variety of resources available for disabled people. You can start by getting in touch with state and local agencies.

Finding Housing

There are many challenges when it comes to finding housing for people with chronic care conditions. In every state, there is a Vocational Rehabilitation Department and most administer housing assistance programs. Other resources include local churches, United Way, and local service organizations working with disabled people, such as centers for the visually impaired. Many people are also turning to social media sites with their needs.

The idea of low-rent apartments probably does not sound too appealing, but you can find places with great neighborhoods, clean surroundings, and friendly people. The government provides funding directly to apartment owners who pass on the savings to renters by lowering the rental rates for low-income tenants. You can find these apartments for disabled, low-income, and seniors. Many are family friendly and pet friendly. You have to pass some requirements such as earn no more than the income limit for the location. You can apply for the rental space by visiting the management office for the apartment complex you are interested in renting. There are other low-rent programs such as housing choice vouchers, public housing, and caregiver homes.

You can look for financial assistance from government agencies. A good place to start is the Department of Housing and Urban Development (HUD). HUD is a government run program which provides a number of programs and maintains a list of approved counseling agencies. In some cases they can provide financial assistance as well. You can reach HUD by calling 800-569-4287 or visiting their website, www.hud.gov. There is a variety of financial assistance for housing and grant programs you can find by going to www.GovBenefits.gov. Here you can research options for housing and financial needs when you are facing disability or chronic care situations.

You can also contact nonprofits in your community. Many community organizations have created national networks that have independent living centers across the United States. With the assistance of necessary accommodations, assistive devices and personal care, independent living is a way for people with disabilities to live on their own and still receive assistance when needed. Before contacting the organizations determine what accommodations you may need.

Everyone with a disability is so different in their needs, some may need a wheelchair ramp and others just financial assistance. There are also group homes available for people with intellectual or psychiatric challenges. You should have a conversation with your providers beforehand to find out what may be required to assist you and your challenges the best way. You can get more information at www.ehow.com/find-housing-disabled-people.

Keeping the Lights On

Benefits for your telephone service are available to low-income clients. It may also be based on availability. You may be eligible for these programs if you are receiving other assistance such as; food stamps, home energy assistance program (HEAP), Medicaid, supplemental security income (SSI), veteran's disability pension (non-service related), or veteran's surviving spouse pension (non-service related).

When you realize that you are going to have trouble paying your utility bills contact the utility company immediately and work out a payment plan. Most companies have programs to help you stretch out your payments based on your income, while they keep your service on. Keep in mind that many of the utility company programs require you to attempt to negotiate a Deferred Payment Agreement (DPA) with your utility before they will accept your application for a payment plan. A Deferred Payment Agreement is a payment schedule that the utility company will create for you based on your income that allows you to pay off your entire bill over time.

When it comes to telephone communications, you can arrange special payment plans, deferred payment plans, quarterly payment plans, and lifeline discounted telephone service. Every telephone communications company offers different plans. I researched Verizon and got the options they had to offer. There are forms that must be filled out to get these arrangements. If on a regular basis you cannot pay your bill by the due date because you are on a fixed income, you may call your service representative to arrange to pay by a different date and late payment charges can be waived. You can apply for a deferred payment plan. This will allow you to retain basic local service while paying past due bills. Plans can be arranged for deferred payment up to $150 for a five-month period through Verizon. If you are disabled because you are a senior (62 or older for Verizon), and your yearly telephone service costs are $150 or less you can arrange to pay quarterly. For adults who are not yet seniors, there is the option of a lifeline-discounted service. This service is offered to disabled people on a fixed income for a reduced rate. This includes the basic monthly charge for telephone service and a discount on installing new services. This option can give you a basic local service at a reduced fee and you can keep the bill even lower by blocking outgoing long distance calls.

There are a few types of lifeline services through telephone companies. Two common ones are message rate service, and flat rate service. For people who are eligible for message rate lifeline services you can pay $1 a month for basic service, plus regional and long-distance fees. This program is best for those who mostly receive calls or who make few calls a month. For people who are eligible for the flat rate life line service you can pay as little as $2 a month for dial tone service charges and you pay a set monthly charge to make unlimited calls within your primary local calling area (as low as $14 per month). Not all of these services are available in all areas so check with your provider. In addition, there may be an installation charge for lifeline service. However, the charge is typically nominal and can be as low as $5 for inside wire and one jack. For more information, call the Life Line Service phone number at 800-799-6874.

Water and Energy Assistance

Every state and utility company offers different programs for assistance with essential utility bills such as water and electricity. Check with the service provider in your area as to which options are available and how to apply for assistance.

In certain circumstances they will assist you with your bills. They can offer you monthly payment agreements to help pay your bills or discounted rates. Some programs can even help you pay for past due bills. There are income guidelines and other qualifications in place and each applicant is screened before assistance is granted. You may not be eligible if you live in subsidized housing and your heat is paid for, if you are a renter/boarder, if you are living in a group home, or if you are living in a temporary housing hotel.

There are a number of different programs available to elderly, disabled, and low-income customers. These programs include deferred payment plans, budget plans, third party notifications, extra security plans, Care and Share plans, and the Neighbor-4-Neighbor Heat Fund. These programs can help those having a hard time making payments or catching up with the amount overdue.

The Deferred Payment plan is for when you have fallen behind on payments and cannot catch up all at once. This plan calls for current bills to be paid on time and in full together with a percentage of the amount overdue until paid.

The Budget plan levels off monthly payments by spreading heating costs over as many as 12 months, making energy bills more predictable and manageable.

The Third Party Notification program allows the customer to designate a relative, friend or agency to receive copies of any termination notice sent to the customer. The third party is not responsible for paying the bill; however, they will become aware of the situation and could possibly offer advice or assistance to the customer to help prevent disconnection of utility service.

The Extra Security plan is for the elderly and permanently disabled. This plan offers an extra measure of security for uninterrupted service. Bill due dates are coordinated to coincide with the arrival of income checks to allow for timely payment. You are eligible if you are 62 years of age or older and retired, or if you are permanently disabled.

The Hospitalized Customer Assistance program provides a 30-day penalty free extension of the bill due date for customers hospitalized for 10 days or more. A physician's statement is necessary to verify the hospital stay.

There are also programs such as Care and Share assistance through the American Red Cross. These applicants must be receiving SSI, SSD, Workers Compensation, or Veterans Disability, elderly, or have a verifiable medical condition that would be directly affected by the loss of electricity (e.g. oxygen machine). Many times the application will require a medical statement from your doctor on their letterhead. Be sure to have your doctor include the condition and state "The absence of electricity or heat will aggravate the patient's condition." In addition to the medical statement you will also need to show proof of age, income, disability (if applicable), picture id, utility bill, and social security number.

There are also great programs such as Neighbor-4-Neighbor Heat Fund run by Catholic Charities and the Salvation Army. This program helps qualified household meet basic and emergency energy needs. You must be disabled, elderly, or have a medical emergency to quality for this program. You can also only apply for one grant, up to $300, per customer, per year.

The Department of Social Services may pay for some of your past-due utility bills depending on your circumstances and if you are on public assistance. Once you get this help, you are typically placed on utility voucher. Although your utilities can still be shut off, under certain circumstances the department will help avoid this from happening. The Department of Social Services may pay the lesser of the four most recent months, or the balance due on the account. In some cases, the applicant will have to sign an agreement to repay the debts within a 12-month period. Even if you are not on public assistance, you may still be eligible for help with your bills; it is always a good idea to check on the possible assistance available to you.

Financial Help for Parents of Disabled Children
There is assistance available for parents with disabled children. Financial assistance can be provided through our federal and state government programs as well as nonprofit organizations. There are dedicated funds through government agencies for children who are disabled.

It is also good to check with disability or disease specific nonprofits that can provide funding, resources, and emotional support for the whole family. The largest federal program is the Social Security Supplemental Income (SSI) to assist families of children with disabilities.

Depending on the condition and varying levels of disability associated with that illness the child may qualify for financial assistance through this program. The program is also based around the financial needs of the child and their family. There is typically a disability evaluation, proof of medical condition, and history of disability requirement associated with this program. You can apply online or by phone with your local SSI office.

There is also temporary emergency assistance for disabled children. The Temporary Assistance for Needy Families or TANF program is available in each state. The state agency is responsible for running its program. This program provides temporary financial assistance to low income families with disabled children. The US Department of Health and Human Services Administration for Children and Families funds this program.

Many nonprofit organizations are dedicated to children with disabilities. Many federal grants are awarded to state agencies and nonprofits. In turn they fund grants to disabled children and their families. Grants do not have to be repaid and are an invaluable option for many families struggling financially because of medical bills to take care of their disabled child. Some grants will pay the difference between insurance coverage and actual health care expenses for the family. There are also grants to individuals for disabled children to obtain equipment such as hearing aids, wheelchairs, eyeglasses, walkers for physical therapy and medical aids.[12]

---

[12] Financial Assistance for Children with Disability Special Needs | Suite101.com www.suite101.com/article/financial-assistance-for-children-with-disability-special-needs

5

DISABILITY RESOURCES

Disability benefits can come from a variety of sources. There is Federal and State assistance for people who are disabled and need financial help. Workman's compensation covers workers injured on the job. Military benefits are available for soldiers and veterans that become disabled while serving our country.

Supplemental Security Income (SSI)

General tax revenues and not Social Security taxes fund the Federal income supplement program. Supplemental Security Income is designed to help aged, blind, and disabled people who have little or no income. It provides cash to meet basic needs for food, clothing, and shelter. You can use the benefits eligibility-screening tool to find out what benefits you qualify to receive.[13]

Typically, if you have a medical condition that has prevented you from working or is expected to prevent you from working for at least 12 months or end in death, you are over 18, and have worked and paid Social Security taxes long enough you will qualify. The more you make (and pay taxes on) and longer you were able to work before disability, the higher your monthly disability check will be. You can apply for disability benefits online or in person at your local office. When you apply online your claim starts immediately as you do not have to wait for an appointment. Being disabled it may be difficult for you to leave your house so the computer process can help you save time, money, and energy.

Medicare

After you receive disability benefits for 24 months, you will be eligible for Medicare. You will get information about Medicare several months

---

[13] www.ssa.gov/pgm/disability.htm

before your coverage starts. I highly suggest that you fill out your papers immediately and return them. Parts of Medicare are free, but additional coverage's are available.

Medicare parts B, C, and D do cost you some of your SSI income each month towards the monthly premium, but it is well worth the money. Medicare part A is free. This is used to help cover inpatient care in hospitals, skilled nursing facilities, hospice, and home health care. Medicare part B helps to cover doctors' services, outpatient care, durable medical equipment, home health services, and other medical services that are deemed medically necessary. Part B also covers some preventive services. Part C is a Medicare Advantage Plan similar to a HMO or PPO. Private companies approved by Medicare offer part C plans. These plans offer extra coverage, such as vision, hearing, dental, and/or health and wellness programs. Most include Medicare prescription drug coverage (Part D). If you do not have a part C that covers medications, you may want to subscribe to Part D. Medicare Part D is prescription drug coverage and is available to everyone with Medicare. To get Part

D, you must join a plan run by an insurance company or other private company approved by Medicare. Each plan can vary in cost and drugs covered.

Keep in mind if you decide not to join a Medicare Parts B, C, or D when you are first eligible, and you do not have other creditable prescription drug coverage, you will likely pay a late enrollment penalty. Check your Medicare card to find out which Parts you are covered under. In addition, if you have permanent kidney failure requiring regular dialysis or a transplant or you have Lou Gehrig's disease, you may qualify for Medicare almost immediately.

If you get Medicare and have low income and few resources, your state may pay your Medicare premiums and, in some cases, other "out-of-pocket" medical expenses such as deductibles and coinsurance. Only your state can decide if you qualify. To find out if you do, contact your state or local welfare office or Medicaid agency. In addition, more information is available from the Centers for Medicare & Medicaid Services by calling Medicare.

Medicaid

There are over 50 million children, families, elderly, and people with disabilities who receive Medicaid benefits assisting with health coverage. This program is available in all 50 states and in most cases is provided at no cost to the recipients. There are different requirements in each state for financial and disability levels. Most state Medicaid programs pay for a full set of services for children. These services including preventive care, immunizations, screening, and treatment of health conditions, doctor visits, hospital visits, and vision and dental care. Depending on the State, you can complete the application through the mail, over the phone, or even on line.

Military Benefits

Military veterans with a service-related disability may qualify for benefits. This type of benefit is paid to veterans who have diseases or injuries that developed while on active duty or were made worse by active military service. These benefits are tax-free and paid to certain veterans who are disabled from Veterans Administration healthcare. Benefits for veterans can include disability pay, travel reimbursement and special compensation for severe disabilities. You are not eligible if you receive a dishonorable discharge. Monthly pay ranges from hundreds to a few thousand dollars. Additional amounts may be paid if you have a loss of limb, have a seriously disabled spouse or you have a dependent (spouse, children, or parents).

You can start the process by filling out the Veterans Application for Compensation or Pension (VA Form 21-526). Follow the instructions on the application and if needed include dependency records and medical evidence. They also offer a wide range of assistance for family members as well. More information can be found on Military benefits in chapter 6.

Other State Assistance Programs

Many states offer specific programs that can help you through daily living. It is important for chronic care patients to maintain independence to sustaining their full range of experiences, rights and desires. Programs that provide training and support appropriate to the needs of each disabled person can be found in every state. You will have to do some digging because the programs vary.

There are a few programs detailed below on food stamps, SSI, Medicaid, and finding other community assistance programs. A good place to start is the office of your local health department. A page of helpful websites can be found in *The Pain Code Journal.*

Food Stamps

Maintaining a healthy balanced diet is very important when you are facing a chronic illness. When your resources are limited, you may be able to qualify for the Supplemental Nutrition Assistance Program. This is a program where you must be qualified to receive assistance. Most applicants and the people in their residence must meet an income limit.

Certain things such as owning a home and vehicles depending on use do not count as income and can be subtracted from your income. Your household may qualify for other income exclusions if it includes a person age 60, older, or disabled. The income limits vary by household size and may change each year. Typically, resources such as cash on hand, in bank accounts and other property are counted towards your available resources. There are other exclusions if the applicant is older than 60 or disabled. All applicants and everyone in your household must have a social security number and be a U.S. citizen, U.S. national or have status as a qualified alien. Applicants, who are healthy and able, between 18-60 years old, must register to work or participate in an employment or training program. In addition, college students may be eligible for assistance.

You can apply for assistance at your local social security office. When you are interviewed at the social security office remember to bring identification, proof of income for each member in your household, proof of childcare expenses, rent or mortgage payment receipts, record of monthly utility charges, and medical bills for disabled or elderly. You can find out how much you may be able to get online through the Supplemental

Nutrition Assistance Program Pre-Screening Tool at www.foodstamps-step1.usda.gov.[14]

Handicap Passes

Handicapped parking is not a fringe benefit of having a chronic illness such as arthritis. It is a necessity for many people living with pain and disability. It is not uncommon for disabled people to wait longer than they should to apply for a handicapped parking placard for their car, which entitles them to park in the designated spots for disabled persons.

Disabled people may not realize at first that they are "eligible". They deny that their condition is debilitating enough to require closer, handicapped parking. They underestimate the benefit of closer parking and how much energy it saves. These passes allow a disabled person to run errands, shop, go to doctor appointments, travel, or participate in other activities, without wearing themselves out within the first few minutes of arriving at their destination.

---

[14] Supplemental Nutrition Assistance Program Facts, www.ssa.gov/pubs/10101.pdf, last modified 5/14/2012

Handicapped parking abusers make it difficult for disabled people. This abuse of handicapped parking permits may also be a disincentive. Too often people who are not entitled to park in handicapped parking spots are found using them. With limited spots available that makes it seem fruitless but it is not. Handicapped parking permits belong in the right hands. People with invisible disabilities (disabilities that do not show outwardly) may fear being mistaken for an abuser of handicapped parking privileges. This group of disabled persons often feels it is not worth being glared at or hassled, yet they are fully entitled to have a handicapped parking permit if their doctor prescribes it.

Getting a Handicapped Parking Placard

If you have a disabling condition which may allow you to have a handicapped parking permit talk to your doctor. Do not wait for your doctor to bring it up to you. Doctors are very busy and it is unlikely that this is foremost on their minds. Your doctor should not hesitate to sign the paperwork for you to get a handicapped parking placard if you are eligible.

Do you know what you need to do to obtain a handicapped parking placard? There are subtle differences between the states regarding what is required. Some states charge a processing fee, while other states offer handicapped parking permits for free. Some states require a doctor's prescription along with an application.

We have compiled the information you need to obtain a handicapped parking permit. Some of the applications for handicapped parking permits can easily be downloaded online.

Alabama - www.revenue.alabama.gov
Arkansas – www.arkansas.gov
California – www.dmv.ca.gov
Colorado - http://driversed.com
Connecticut - www.ct.gov
Delaware - www.dmv.de.gov
Florida - www.hsmv.state.fl.us
Georgia - www.dds.ga.gov
Hawaii - www.state.hi.us
Idaho - http://itd.idaho.gov
Iowa - www.iadotforms.dot.state.ia.us
Illinois - www.sos.state.il.us
Indiana - www.in.gov
Kansas - www.ksrevenue.org
Kentucky - www.ecclix.com

Louisiana - https://web01.dps.louisiana.gov
Massachusetts - www.mass.gov
Maryland- http://mva.state.md.us
Maine - www.maine.gov
Michigan - www.michigan.gov
Missouri - www.dor.mo.gov
Mississippi - www.mstc.state.ms.us
Montana - www.doj.mt.gov
North Carolina - www.ncdot.org
North Dakota - www.dot.nd.gov
Nebraska - www.dmv.state.ne.us
New Hampshire - www.nh.gov
New Jersey - www.state.nj.us
New Mexico - www.tax.state.nm.us
Nevada - www.dmvnv.com
New York - www.nydmv.state.ny.us
Ohio - www.bmv.ohio.gov
Oklahoma - http://driversed.com
Oregon - www.oregon.gov
Pennsylvania - www.dmv.state.pa.us
Rhode Island - www.dmv.ri.gov
South Carolina - www.scdmvonline.com
South Dakota - www.state.sd.us
Tennessee - www.state.tn.us
Texas - www.dot.state.tx.us
Utah - http://dmv.utah.gov
Virginia -http://www.dmv.state.va.us
Vermont - http://dmv.vermont.gov
Washington - http://www.dol.wa.gov
Washington D.C. - http://dmv.dc.gov
Wisconsin - www.dot.wisconsin.gov
West Virginia - www.wvdmv.gov
Wyoming - www.dot.state.wy.us

Bus Passes

I used to take the bus often. Make sure to learn the schedule and let the bus driver know if you have any disabilities or need any assistance. Ask him to remind you to get off the bus at your final destination or transfer location. Get a bus pass for disabled riders. They are available in most states and typically give you free or discounted rides. Some cities have vans that the disabled can call for special pickups so that you are not on the crowded bus. This comes in handy when you have a pain condition and it is rough on you to be bumped or stepped on which can happen on a crowded bus.

Transportation to your doctor visits

Patient transportation services are available for patients. These services are available to Medicaid and Workers Compensation insured patients. These companies ensure that patients are transported with the right level of medical expertise in the most appropriate vehicle (specialty vans accommodating wheelchairs) in order to meet the patient's healthcare needs in an economical manner. Modes of transport include ambulatory, wheelchair, stretcher, and air ambulance.

Typically, the company will contact the patient to ensure a smooth transition from home to their appointments and back. The company will report non-compliant claimants and missed appointments to the Case Managers or Claims Adjusters within the hour to assist with the rescheduling of appointments. This will allow immediate intervention to prevent lapse of recovery or possible re-injury. Most will call patients the night before pickup to make sure the service is still needed. The insurance company is directly billed with a detailed invoice as to miles driven, time of transport, and drop off locations. Some companies are able to provide multi-lingual staff. Services are typically available everyday of the year. You can set up this service with your claims adjuster or care manager.

Walking Through the Minefield of the Health System

6

INSURANCE

Health insurance is insurance against the risk of incurring medical expenses that are catastrophic. Although I cannot imagine a time with no medical insurance for society, this type of insurance did not develop into the model we have today until the middle to late 20th century. People paid the cost of seeing the doctor or getting emergency care out of their own pocket. This was known as a fee-for-service business model.

We now rely on a medical insurance system that provides comprehensive programs that cover a range of needs such as routine, preventive, and emergency health procedures. Most insurance companies also cover prescribed medications to some extent. However, it was not until the 1920's that individual hospitals began to offer medical services to patients on a pre-paid basis, leading to the development of Blue Cross organizations.[15] Now there are multiple plan types available depending on the situation that you need coverage or protection. Plans are administered by organizations such as a government agency, private business, or not-for-profit entities.

In 2006, PricewaterhouseCoopers released a study which examined the cause of rising health care costs in the United States. This study pointed to increased consumption created by increased consumer demand, new treatments, and more intensive diagnostic testing, as the most significant.[16] This may or may not have affected the outcome of the study but it should be noted that after the study was released, Wendell Potter, a long-time PR representative for the health insurance industry, noted that the group which sponsored the study, AHIP, is a front-group funded by various insurance companies.[17]

---

[15] Fundamentals of Health Insurance: Part A, Health Insurance Association of America, 1997, ISBN 1-879143-36-4
[16] The Factors Fueling Rising Healthcare Costs 2006, PricewaterhouseCoopers for America's Health Insurance Plans, 2006
[17] Deadly Spin: An Insurance Company Insider Speaks Out on How Corporate PR is Killing Health Care and Deceiving Americans, 2010, pg.205

Other factors caused the increase in medical treatment options. There has been a movement for plans that provide a broader array of options, high-tech technologies, and the cost shifting from Medicaid patients and under or noninsured to the private paying population. [14]   Another cause of healthcare price increases is that we are living longer especially in developed countries.

As our population ages a larger population of citizens requires more intensive medical care than the younger population. There have also been great advances in medicine and health technology. As new diagnostic machines, medications, and lifesaving tools are developed with such complexity, the cost of the treatment options available also increases. There has also been an increase in population size, followed by unhealthy life choices such as alcohol abuse, smoking, people not exercising as much, and the increased use of street drugs. Finally, providers are often times incentivized for treating patients rather than curing patients and patients who are insured with good coverage will go to the best providers who are typically the more expensive providers.[18]

The healthcare system relies on private health insurance as coverage for most Americans, and most providers bill the insurance company directly if the patient signs an agreement that say they are responsible if the insurance company does not pay. Whether you have private health insurance or are on a public program it is important to know your coverage limits and fees associated with your plan.

Medical Insurance

When comparing medical insurance plans be sure to pay attention to the entire written statement. Deciding on which plan to choose, can be confusing. You should breakdown the technical jargon and see how each policy varies, and which is best for you. The cheapest is not always the worst policy and the most expensive does not necessarily cover all of the care you may need. If you are in the process of deciding between

---

[18] Robert E. Wright, Fubarnomics: A Lighthearted, Serious Look at America's Economic Ills (Buffalo, N.Y.: Prometheus, 2010)

enrolling in a HMO, PPO, Catastrophic, or POS you can often compare the plans by going online to the insurance companies' website that will be providing the coverage to learn about the benefits and costs of each plan.

Health Maintenance Organizations / HMO

Health Maintenance Organizations offer health plans, which refer to a subscription-based medical care arrangement. HMOs are comprised of hospitals, doctors and associated medical personnel who have contracted to provide healthcare to members in return for a pre-paid monthly medical insurance charge. When you elect to join an HMO health plan, you select a doctor as your "primary care physician" (PCP) from a list provided by the HMO.

Typically, family practitioners, internists, and pediatricians manage all medical care including referrals to specialists and determining whether further lab tests or x-rays are needed. This can be a good situation to be in because having a lead doctor who must coordinate with your other doctors is a benefit to the patient and can eliminate any unnecessary care. The drawback comes when you would like to see a specialist or get a second opinion and have to get a referral to do so. If your PCP does not agree with you, it may be difficult to obtain and then you would have to pay out of pocket for additional services.

The plan typically pays for a fixed number of services: for instance, a certain number of days of hospice care, a fixed number of home health visits, a fixed number of chiropractic session, etc. There is usually a review person contracted by the HMO and it is at their discretion as to the services offered to you. This part of the process can occur prior to or after hospital admission.

The basics of an HMO plan:
- All of the providers in the HMO network are required to file a claim to get paid
- Except for certain types of care that may not be available from a network provider, you must choose doctors, hospitals, and other providers in the HMO network, or your care is not covered

- Hospital expenses are usually covered at 100% for little or no copays
- In order to see a doctor for an office visit, you would pay a small copays - usually $10 or $15
- Plans are available on both a group and individual basis
- Prescriptions are available for a small copays
- The only charges you should incur for in-network services are copayments for doctor's visits and other services such as procedures and prescriptions
- This type of plan was formed with the idea of controlling costs by providing preventative healthcare
- You will need a referral from your primary care physician to see a specialist (such as a neurologist or surgeon) except in emergencies
- Your HMO will not provide coverage if you do not have a primary care physician and this PCP must refer you to a specialist who is in the HMO network

Preferred Provider Organizations / PPO

Preferred Provider Organizations offer health insurance that has contracts with a network of "preferred" providers you can choose. You do not have to have a referral to see a specialist or select a designated PCP. This can make it easier for you to get to the correct provider who knows about your specific condition. When you receive care from a doctor in the preferred network, you will only be responsible for your annual deductable and a copayment for your visit.

When you use an out-of-network provider to get health services, you will pay a higher amount of copayment. For example, if the out-of-network doctor charged you $100 for a visit, you are responsible for the full amount if you have not met your deductable. If you have met the deductable, the PPO pays a percentage and you will pay the rest of the bill. Typically after the deductable is met this is covered 60/40% or 50/50%. This encourages you to use providers who have a negotiated price with the insurance company, saving them money as well as yourself.

The basics of a PPO plan:
- If you get your healthcare from a network provider, you usually do not need to file a claim
- If you go out of network for services, you may have to pay the provider in full and then file a claim with the PPO to be reimbursed and the money you receive from the PPO will most likely be only part of the bill
- When using an out of network provider, you are responsible for any part of the doctor's fee that the PPO does not pay
- In most PPO networks, you will only be responsible for the copayment. (Some PPO's do have an annual deductable for any services, in network or out of network)
- You can choose doctors, hospitals, and other providers from the PPO network or from out-of-network. If you choose an out-of-network provider, you most likely will pay more
- You do not need a referral to see a specialist but some specialists will only see patients who are referred to them by a primary care doctor

- Some PPO's require that you get a prior approval for certain expensive services, such as MRIs

High Deductable Plan /HDP

There are a growing number of employers and employees turning to high-deductable plans (HDP), which is considered coverage in catastrophic situations. These are plans that are used in the purpose of catastrophic care. They offer the patient lower monthly premiums in exchange for higher deductibles. Many of these plans are paired with health savings accounts (HSA's) which help pay for qualified care and medications, but not all high-deductible health plans can be paired with an HSA.

When you have a HDP expect to pay for all of your medical expenses, until your percentage of medical expenses has been reached for the year. Some plans will then pay up to 100 percent of the medical bills for that year after you reach your out-of-pocket maximum. Just as with other types of insurance, your monthly premiums do not count toward your deductible or your out-of-pocket maximum.

It is not unusual to see the out-of-pocket costs at over $5,000 a year. This could be a good plan if you are hardly sick, injured, or do not have a chronic health condition. Alternatively, if you have a secondary insurance such as Medicare to assist with the out-of-pocket costs this may be a good choice for you.

A health savings account lets you set aside pre-tax money to use for medical care today or in future retirement. For a HDP to qualify to be paired with your HSA, certain criteria must be met. The plan must have a deductible of at least $1,200 for an individual and $2,400 for a family and the out-of-pocket maximums can be no more than $5,950 for an individual and $11,900 for a family. There is a maximum you can contribute tax free to your account each year; $3,050 per individual, up to $6,150 as a family.

If you are 55 or older, you can save an additional $1,000 per year. As long as the withdraws are for qualified medical expenses (deductable, medical not covered by your plan, dental or vision expenses) you do not have to pay taxes on them. There is a tax penalty incurred if you use the funds from your HSA on non-medical expenses and you are not yet 65 years old or older. A good part of the HSA account is that even if you change employers or health plans, the money is still yours to spend on healthcare.

Be sure you completely understand your health insurance options. If you are considering a catastrophic plan, make sure you understand how the plan works, what it covers and how much you might end up paying out of pocket. Otherwise, you may run into a situation where you owe thousands of dollars in deductibles and copayments and your insurance company ends up paying little to nothing towards your bills. One plan I was almost suckered into would have cost me $5,000 per medical event, so if I had undergone multiple hospital stays in that year, the cost could have been astronomically catastrophic for me. Luckily, I realized the issue within an hour of signing up for this policy and was able to cancel.

Secondary Insurance

It can be very beneficial financially to have secondary insurance such as Medicare when your primary plan has a very high deductable. Essentially your secondary insurance will pick up what the primary coverage will not, therefore, covering most or all of your deductable. This can be very helpful financially.

Point of Service Plan / POS

A Point-of-Service plan has combined the features of an HMO and PPO and is a type of managed-care health insurance system. However, POS health insurance does differ from other managed care plans. When the patient enrolls in a POS plan, they are required to choose an in-network primary care physician to monitor the patient's health care. This PCP becomes their "point of service" provider. The primary POS physician may then make referrals outside the network, but then only some compensation may be offered by the patient's health insurance company.

Dental Insurance

Good dental hygiene is important for our overall health. Being able to get dental care should be high on our priority list. Insurance is available to assist with costs associated with dental care. As with health insurance, there are several types of dental insurance: individual; family; or group.

Dental insurance plans fall into three categories: Preferred Provider Networks; Dental Health Managed Organizations; and Indemnity Dental Insurance. There are also basic and major procedures. Coverage will depend on the type of procedure the patient is having. Basic procedures often include fillings, periodontics, endodontics, and oral surgery. Major procedures often are crowns, dentures, and implants. Procedures such as periodontics, endodontics, and oral surgery may fall into the major procedure category depending on your specific plan with specific fee schedules and co-payments.

Depending on your specific plan, if you seek an Out-of-Network or Non-Participating Provider, any difference of fees will become the financial responsibility of the patient unless otherwise specified in your dental policy.

Keep in mind that many dental insurance plans may have waiting periods no matter which type of plan you are covered under. Generally, this waiting period is set in place before you are enrolled in a plan and it sets a schedule of maintenance visits before certain benefits will be covered. For example, the patient must wait six months between cleanings, or getting x-rays every two years for the service to be covered.

Some dental insurance plans may have a yearly maximum benefit limit. Once the maximum benefit is exhausted for that year, additional treatments may become the patient's responsibility. Each year that annual maximum is reissued. So when needed, I would schedule my dental work in December and January to take most benefit of the coverage. Keep in mind that your coverage may have a different anniversary date. When possible, plan your dental work around the policy to ensure you get the most coverage from your plan

When it comes to Orthodontics, policies usually have separate annual deductible depending on the type of treatment rendered. After the patient pays the yearly deductible, the remaining dental plan benefit is paid at its specified fee schedule.

Preferred Provider Network Dental plans / DPPN:

- Dental insurance companies have fee schedules based on usual and customary dental services
- Fee schedules are established on an average of providers fees in your area
- When a dentist signs a contract with a dental insurance company that provider agrees to match the insurance companies fee schedule and give their customers a reduced cost for services

Dental Health Managed Organizations /DHMO:

- The patient is assigned to an in-network dentist or in-network dental office and must stay within that network to receive the dental benefits

Indemnity Plan /DIP:

- These plans allow you to see any dentist you want who accepts insurance

Explanation of Benefits (EOB)

As with medical claims processed through an insurance company, the patient will receive an Explanation of Benefits (EOB) statement after services are delivered to the patient. The EOB papers are most often sent with payment to the provider of service and a second copy of the papers are sent to the patient.

I always compare my EOB to my provider's bill. Many times the EOB states I owe a lot less than the doctor bill, or in some cases, I owe nothing at all. In the event the explanation of benefits does not match the doctor bill, I make a copy of the EOB, highlighting where it says "patients responsibility", and pay only that amount. When I have done this, I have never received another doctor bill for that service as the provider updates their system with the EOB information I provided.

Military Health Coverage

The health care program for Uniformed Service members, retirees and their families is Tricare insurance. Eligibility is determined by the Uniformed Services and then reported to the Defense Enrollment Eligibility Reporting System (DEERS). Tricare offers a variety of plans. Depending on your military status, you may not have a monthly premium for your care.

There is also a Tricare dental and vision program available for some service members and their families. In cases where a service member would like to see a provider that is not in the Tricare network, you must request a waiver from the TRICARE Overseas Program (TOP) contractor. If a waiver is granted for an episode, after the episode is complete you must return to using a Tricare provider to continue care or your claim may be denied.

In 2012, there are eight plans offered:
- Tricare Prime Options (TPO)
- Tricare for Life (TFL)
- Tricare Standard and Extra (TSE)

- Tricare Standard Overseas (TSO)
- Tricare Reserve Select (TRS)
- Tricare Retired Reserve (TRR)
- Tricare Young Adult (TYA)
- US Family Health Plan (USFHP)

Plans cost $0.00 to $1,024.43 per month for the annual premium. Costs are dependent on if you purchase it as an individual or have a family, and under which plan you qualify. Premiums are adjusted annually, but you may purchase Tricare coverage at anytime throughout the year.

Some plans have additional coverage requirements. An example is if you are entitled to Medicare and are not an active duty family member, by law you must be enrolled and pay Medicare Part B premiums to remain eligible for Tricare.

Different federal laws govern Medicare and Tricare, therefore each program determines the specific medical services it covers. There are situations in which Medicare will pay for some services that Tricare does not cover and vice versa. Typically, Medicare is billed first and Tricare will pay the balance on the Medicare claim leaving the policyholder no out-of-pocket expense for the services on that claim.

According to the Tricare website, a vast majority of TFL claims are like this. In a case where one policy covers the service received and the other does not, the covering policy will pay its portion and the patient is responsible for the remaining service and deductible costs. [19]

Workers Compensation

When an employee is injured on the job, there is insurance that may cover them instead of the regular medical insurance policy. This insurance is known as Workers Compensation or Work Comp. The first work comp law in the United States was passed in 1902 by the state of Maryland and the federal law was passed in 1906.[20] By 1949, all states had enacted workers' compensation laws.[21] The WC insurance can replace lost wages and

---

[19] Tricare forms, visit www.tricare.mil/mybenefit/home

[20] loislaw.com, The Employers Liability Cases, 207 U.S. 463, 1908

[21] lawphil.net, The Employers' Liability Act of Alabama, first enacted in 1855 (Civil Code 1907, Ch. 80, sec. 3910), is a substantial, if not an exact copy, of the English Act of 1880

provide medical benefits. This is done in exchange for mandatory surrender of the employee's right to sue his or her employer for the tort of negligence.

This is a tradeoff of coverage, because you as a patient accepting WC insurance payments will be limited on coverage and lack recourse if the WC adjusters are unwilling to work with you. Although in the United States injured employees have a right to medical care for the injury, work comp companies still have a hand in what treatments they will cover, what doctors you can see, and what medications you can take. If you do not choose to follow what the Work Comp Company chooses for you, you will be responsible for the cost of care incurred.

I have a few friends who have gone through this process, one in particular for over 20 years. Every few years she ends up back in court or having to threaten to go to court to get medical bills covered. The laws in each state differ as well as the allowances of specific plans and adjusters.

Coverage can be gained for payments in place of wages, economic losses, medical expenses, and benefits payable to the employee's dependants when killed during employment. Compensation for negligence, pain/suffering, and punitive damages is generally not available as a part of a work comp case. The amount of compensation is based on the types of injury sustained, the job skills of the now disabled employee, and if the person is able to find employment in partial capacity.

The statutes do not account for the difficulty in finding work that is suitable for the disabled employee. In addition, caps on the value of the loss/ disability do not always reflect the total cost of providing for the disabled employee. Compensation can be far less than the amount required to keep a person in reasonable living conditions for the remainder of their life.

Dealing with a work comp case can be very stressful because some employers vigorously contest employee claims for workers' compensation payments. Any case that is contested or a severe injury has occurred should be overseen by a well-versed lawyer with specific work comp experience, instead of the disabled employee.

When an employer protests payment for a work related injury, it comes down to financials. Many states have laws that limit a claimant's legal expenses to a certain fraction of an award (11%-40%).[22] Disputes may be handled in court or informally by administrative law judges. Appeals may be brought up to an appeals board, and if not resolved, into the court system. The point of worker compensation was to reduce litigation, but a few states still allow the disabled employee to initiate a lawsuit in a trial court.[23] If you are going through a work comp case be ready for the stress, anxiety and pressure the process is bound to bring onto your already unsolicited challenges of being disabled on the job.

Health Insurance Terms

- Capitation: A fee paid by an insurer to a provider, for which the provider agrees to treat all members of the insurer

---

[22] A Study of Nonsubscription to the Texas Workers' Compensation System: 2001, Joseph Shields and D. C. Campbell, www.iaiabc.org/files/public/Texas%20-%20Research.pdf

[23] California Workers' Compensation Claims and Benefits, by Judge David W. O'Brien, JudgeOBrien.com

- Coinsurance: Instead of, or in addition to, paying a fixed amount up front (co-payment), the co-insurance is a percentage of the total cost that the insured person might also have to pay
- Co-payment: The amount that the insured person must pay out of pocket before the health insurer pays for a particular service
- Coverage limits: The health plan will stop payment when they reach the benefit maximum, and the policy-holder must pay all remaining costs
- Deductible: The amount that the insured must pay out-of-pocket before health insurer pays
- Exclusions: The insured are generally expected to pay the full cost of non-covered services out of their own pockets
- Explanation of Benefits: A document that may be sent by an insurer to a patient explaining what was covered for a medical service
- In-Network Provider: Generally, providers in-network are providers who have a contract with the insurer to accept rates further discounted from the "usual and customary" charges the insurer pays to out-of-network providers

- Out-of-pocket maximums: Similar to coverage limits, except that in this case, the insured person's payment obligation ends when they reach the out-of-pocket maximum, and health insurance pays all further covered costs
- Premium: The amount the policy-holder or their sponsor (e.g. an employer) pays to the health plan to purchase health coverage
- Prior Authorization: An authorization that an insurer provides prior to medical service occurring

Challenges with Insurance

Americans receive their health care coverage from a variety of sources through employment, self-purchased, and public programs such as Medicare. As the costs of new high-tech healthcare and machines dramatically rise consumers have seen a significant hike in premiums, out-of-pocket costs for deductibles, copayments, and other cost sharing.

Insurance companies are also working to keep their operation costs down. Insurers are doing this through policies such as prior authorization practices, step therapy requirements, and specialty tier pricing on medications.

Appealing Decisions

It can be a battle that is time consuming, frustrating, and depressing when an insurance company denies a medication, procedure or durable medical equipment. Sometimes the issue is due to a provider entering the wrong code but most often it is a cost savings issue with the insurance companies. They can question whether a certain treatment is appropriate for someone with your condition. This is done generically and it is important to appeal these decisions.

By doing blanket denials an insurance company can save a lot of money. Many patients and providers give up when they get the first denial letter. An appeal can show a pattern that other patients with the same condition also need the same treatment and that it is beneficial for your condition. This can lead to an easier situation for other patients down the line, as well as if you need the procedure repeated, like in the case of booster infusions.

If you receive a denial letter from your provider, begin your appeal by first figuring out what led to the denial of coverage. Research your insurance company's procedures for an appeal. Some allow phone calls others have a mountain of paperwork for you and your provider to complete. When you call your insurance provider, it is important to take notes, including the name of who you spoke with and the date and time. Include this information on your appeal letter. You can find the detailed guidelines on the insurer's website or in the Evidence of Coverage book that your employer or Medicare sent you at the start of your coverage period. Knowing what their guidelines and policies are for a specific condition or treatment option can be beneficial in writing your appeal.

Understand your plans benefits and rules as your access to this treatment option my hinge on you proving your treatment qualifies for coverage. Other issues can be involved such as if your insurance company feels that the treatment is proven and medically necessary. Sometimes including documents and recent studies showing effectiveness can go a long way with getting access to coverage. You can ask your provider to write a detailed letter on your behalf.

If you are able, work on a draft copy so it takes the provider less time, and they will be more willing to help. You will also want to get a copy of your medical records that pertain to this condition/procedure and send a copy of those as well. I like to highlight key points in my records to ensure it is more likely the appeals board sees specific information when making a final decision. Sometimes it takes multiple appeals to get the treatment option passed.

When looking for studies and documents that demonstrate that the treatment you wish to have insurance cover be sure to use strong publications. Look for studies that included large, randomized, controlled trials. Nevertheless, anything published could help your case. If you are not sure, you can ask your provider to explain the parts of the study that you do not understand to make sure the study or research article is appropriate.

If you come to a point of exhaustion with your insurance companies appeal process, you may want to try for your state's appeals process when your insurance is through your employer or individual policy. Every state has its own rules as to whether or not your case qualifies for appeal at this level. If you contact your state insurance regulation office they will be able to guide you in the appropriate direction. For those who are on Medicare there is a separate appeals process that is run federally and you can start the appeals process at www.medicare.gov. Use state and federal appeals as a last resort and remember that not all situations qualify through these so you have to check with the state regulator or Medicare for additional information if you reach this level of appeal need.

Step Therapy / Fail First

There are big efforts from patient organizations and advocates to stop the "fail first" or "step therapy" practices to biologics and other drugs. However, insurance companies continue to apply practice in an effort to save them money. There are patients from all over the United States reporting how they are being forced to switch from one drug to another. This has personally happened to me twice. Both times, I fought the ruling using my medical records and providers support and the insurance company reversed the decision. However, others are not so lucky. In my case, I had already tried all of the medications that the insurance company was willing to pay for. I had documented records stating my reaction to each of the medications.

On this most recent incident my doctor also filed Voluntary Medform 3500 on my behalf which was one of the requirements by the insurance company as part of my appeal. This process can be overwhelming, detrimental to your health, and time consuming if you have not already tried the medications they are now requiring. Even for me it took two months of calls, paperwork, and appeals to achieve a positive outcome. When you have a chronic condition, this fail first policy will force the patient to prove to the insurance company that another, often less effective treatment has failed to work before allowing them to move onto another option. In some cases, the patient has been on the correct medication for years when they receive their notice that they must try a less expensive, often less effective medication.

In my case, I had to prove that the other medications failed to work before my insurer would be willing to cover the medication my provider had me on and was proven effective in helping me. Simply, this undermines the patient-provider relationship that is vital to assuring the best medical outcomes for the patient. This type of measure might save insurance companies in the short term, but long-term health issues, increases to the ER and hospital due to complications only increase the insurer's costs overtime. There needs to be an open dialogue with insurance companies to draw attention to the adverse affects on such policies affecting the patient's life and treatment outcomes.

We need to abolish the unethical "Step Therapy" or "Fail First" practices by insurance plans. There are legislative efforts in many states that would prohibit a health plan from using step therapy when a physician has prescribed a medication. These efforts seek to prohibit or limit plans from requiring a patient to use a different medication than the one prescribed by the patient's physician.

Usually, a patient can tell immediately whether a medication is working or not and they should not be forced to stay on medicine which does not relieve symptoms. Applying step therapy protocols rigidly to a chronic care patient is not in the patient's best interest and simply creates undue challenges to pain patients. This practice is especially hard on pain patients who are women, minorities, and economically disadvantaged patients. Studies have shown these groups are most affected and are either disproportionately undertreated or go untreated for pain. We must urge insurers to reduce health disparities in our communities.

If you are faced with a step therapy situation, what can you do? I would suggest you appeal immediately. If you have already tried that medication get copies of your providers' records, and your journal entries and submit them with the appeal. You can use your journal to help the provider find the records for the correct dates of services where adverse affects were reported. If you are in a state that allows for step therapy practices to occur be sure to document each day and step of the new medication in your journal. Note as soon as complications and bad side effects occur and report it to your doctor. You should also have your provider fill out and submit voluntary Medform 3500 that when you do have a bad reaction or a medication is not helping. Then, if you are ever in a situation, it will already be documented and chances of successful appeal are favorable to you.

Prior Authorizations

There are some insurance plans that require prior authorization (PA) requests from your provider for specific medication for you. Your insurance plan may not provide coverage or pay for your medication if you do not get this prior approval. Typically, this PA requirement is for expensive medications and medications that treat chronic illnesses. Once again, this tactic is used as a cost containment measure. The insurance provider will only pay for medical treatment, service, medications, and procedures that have been approved in advance. The patient must go through the PA process to obtaining approval from a private or public third-party prescription insurer. The process covers the correctness, suitability, and coverage of a service or medication that allows a beneficiary to know in advance about whether their request will be covered under their plan.

The process differs with each plan but is supposed to ensure that a patient will receive the appropriate level of care in the appropriate setting. This is actually a technique for minimizing costs, wherein benefits are only paid if the medical care has been pre-approved. It can delay care months to years, and can be life threatening and health deteriorating to the patient, in many ways.

Services that may require prior authorization requests:

- All inpatient admissions
- Back surgery
- Hysterectomies
- Maternity stays longer than 48 hours
- Non-childbirth observation stays
- Potentially cosmetic procedures

- Potentially experimental and investigational procedures
- Some outpatient procedures

Specialty Tier

Insurance companies have divided medications and treatments into four main insurance tiers based on type and price. The top and most expensive tier is known as the "specialty tier" or "tier 4 medications". Insurance companies classify the most innovative, expensive, and most essential to life medications as specialty tier. The specialty tier medications are costing patients hundreds to thousands of dollars each month. Patients with chronic care diseases such as arthritis, Reflex Sympathetic Dystrophy, Hemophilia, HIV/ AIDS, Crohn's disease, Hepatitis C, Multiple Sclerosis, and many forms of cancer struggle to afford the medication they need to keep them functioning on a daily basis.[24]

According to the National Minority Quality Forum, 57 million Americans depend on specialty

---

[24] Specialty Tier drugs,
www.managedcaremag.com/archives/0903/0903.formfiles.html

drugs. Tier 4 specialty drugs provide treatment for the chronic care population. These drugs are typically expensive and with no generic form yet available. They also may require special handling or administration to the patient. By 2010, specialty tier drugs increased in price by 19.6%, versus the 1.4% increase for traditional drugs. It is projected by 2013 that specialty tier drug prices are expected to increase 27.5%.[25]

With specialty tier pricing, a patient pays a co-insurance instead of a copays, so instead of a normal cost, the cost out of pocket for the patient can become astronomical. This is done to patients who are typically disabled or classified as needing catastrophic care and low-income patients. It is difficult to appeal this type of tier system as medications are classified and a list available to the insured at the time of coverage or when a medication is released to the market.

---

[25] Specialty tiers: unequal treatment, 2010, National Minority Quality Forum, www.nmqf.org/IB3SpecialtyTiersFinal.pdf

Walking Through the Minefield of the Health System

7

REACH OUT

Reach out to other patients in your area and online. Often times, your health care professionals do not have time to give you the everyday in's and out's of your condition. Speaking with and learning from people who have been through what you are now facing can be a great way to lessen your daily struggles. Not only should you reach out as a patient but your family, friends, and caregivers on your team should also reach out to others in similar situations.

It can be quite difficult to live alone and the struggles only increase when you must leave the house because of chronic illness or disability. Often time patients isolate themselves and go days without seeing or speaking to anybody. This can lead to severe depression and anxiety. Chronically ill or disabled patients are vulnerable to social isolation. There are many free support groups and services in your community. All you have to do is reach out and ask for assistance.

Teaming up with a non-disabled person can help you to be more involved in the community and can improve your quality of life. You can set up telephone safety checks where people have specific times to call you and make sure you are okay and give you some social stimulation. You can ask for practical assistance such as someone preparing your food for the week ahead of time so that you can keep proper nutrition. Join social clubs in person or online to encourage you to keep moving and remind you to do your physical therapy exercises each day. Set up a monthly trip to keep you socializing and give you something to look forward to instead of doctor's appointments all the time. It can be something as simple as going for ice cream or a movie. Having a team of advocates to assist you can make your life easier to live.

Reaching out helps patients integrate into mainstream society. Instead of being disabled, people can see you as a person with different abilities. I joke that my husband does all of the physical activities (yard work, cooking, bathing me) and I stick to the mental activities (paying bills, keeping organized, keeping track of doctor appointments, and when an oil change is needed).

Make it a Family Affair

So many lifestyle changes come with a chronic condition. You can make your life easier if you develop a plan of action and set the expectation with your family in the early stages of your chronic condition. Invite family members and friends to join you in your planning and learning about the challenges that will be faced as a chronic care patient. Doing it together can keep everyone on the same page and working smarter instead of harder.

Your caregivers and loved ones can help you negotiate the complex healthcare and education system. They can be your voice when you are not up to the challenge of specific situations. By accepting help when needed you can build your abilities to help yourself. Taking the help can give you more energy to spend on other activities and situations that will go undone otherwise. Your support team members can provide guidance, family empowerment and appropriate help. That is why it is important to include them in your care decisions and in setting expectations as soon as you can. This is a great way to keep it a family experience instead of a family fight.

Today, more than ever, families are dependent on other people and the community. As society has become more complex, families often are far away from relatives who can be counted on to help in chronic care situations. It is common for all adults in the family to work. So often times it leaves the disabled patient at home alone to fend for themselves. Going to community resources for diagnosis and treatment of health problems, financial aid, childcare, parent education, medical information, referral hotlines, legal assistance, and recreation services can help a patient thrive and overcome challenges. When resources are hard to find you must make an effort to find out what is available in your community. Use all resources available to you including local government, churches, schools, nonprofit organizations, and healthcare providers. Check with employers for support with flexible work hours, part-time work, and time off for assisting the disabled or ill patient.

Finding Community

From time to time, we all need help. Most families will face a health crisis with at least one family member at some point. Just as children need the support of families, families need the support of society. Often times, even when services are available people do not like to use them. They feel they are a burden, or it is meant for someone "worse off than me". They may see help as a sign of weakness. I have a family member who has multiple sclerosis. When she comes to visit, she feels asking one of us to take her to the doctor for her weekly shot is a burden. She would rather go with no medication and suffer the pain and loss of energy then be a burden. What she is not seeing is that her poor health takes a bigger toll on the family. We cannot solve all problems on our own and by asking for assistance from our community members and family does not make us a burden.

Asking for help shows you care about yourself and your loved ones. When you seek out and accept help it allows you to have an advantage over your challenges. As a patient you benefit from the support of your community. You may feel less isolated and more a part of your community. Working with others can enable you to grow personally and learn what you have to offer to others. In addition, it is always helpful to know that other people have similar problems. You can strengthen your family and friends when you use local services and opportunities available to you.

Make every effort to find out what services are available in your area and make use of them. Do your part to urge society to meet its responsibility to the people who need chronic care due to illness or disability. Knowing about these services can improve the quality of life for you, your family, and your caregivers. You may be surprised at how many people there are ready to help you and your family.

For child sitting services contact colleges, high schools, friends, women's organizations, relatives, and neighbors. This comes in handy especially when I am under anesthesia and my husband has to work. It is not just for children and pets. For leisure activities on a budget contact movie theaters, sports teams, support groups, recreation departments, museums, sports clubs, community pools, YMCA, or YWCA for discounts.

For single parent groups you can contact Parents Without Partners (PWP), Big Brothers/Big Sisters, or singles clubs. As a child of a single mother, I found PWP activities great and never knew how little my mom paid for us to participate in great experiences that gave me memories of a lifetime.

For healthcare on a budget, contact your local health department or hospital. Ask about dental exams, checkups for eyes, speech, hearing, chest exams, and mental health services. For counseling services contact churches, hotlines, clinics, or family service agencies.

Support Groups

There are many reasons support groups are valuable to the individuals who create and maintain them. Support groups can be a great experience if you find a group that is positive and the leaders are open to different philosophies of managing your condition, as we know not everything works for every patient. In a good support group individuals who share like problems or situations work together to understand and/ or improve their situations. These members own and operate the group. This offers participants experiential knowledge, information, education, and emotional support. Typically, the group leaders are not paid and are members or starters of the group. For the members participation is free or there might be a small charge for special group activities. There are support groups for most conditions, as well as groups that encompass multiple conditions, with a focus on all pain or neuropathy pain conditions. Many of the groups grow to provide educational materials and advocacy to the community.[26]

Many times a group's accomplishments far exceed those of the medical profession and can provide individual patients support for everyday living. There can be great power with support group initiatives to raise self-advocacy. There is great value to be gained by mutual support from individuals going through similar situations where you find yourself. To find a local support group you can do a search on Google, supportgroups.com, meetup.com, or check with your providers and local hospitals.

The positive sides of joining a support group:
- Empathy from others going through what you are challenged by
- Experiential options may be discussed and relief may be found through these other means
- Members can share their challenges and solutions to challenges others might also face with the same condition

---

[26] Self Help Movement, www.answers.com/topic/self-help-movement

- Members grow their own personal understanding as they share their stories
- Raising awareness and advocacy in the communities the members live in, helping establish an understanding of their specific condition
- Social bonds may form, helping members to establish a new network of friends who have like problems
- Support groups offer information and education about specific problems or situations faced by its members, and how to deal with them
- You can get a different perspective from what you get from the healthcare providers view

The Negative side of support groups
- Less personal interaction
- People sometimes confuse the meaning of something they read verses hearing it directly from the person and being able to see the context in which it is meant
- You must have access to a computer and know how to use it to be able to participate

Online self-help groups offer their own sets of benefits and drawbacks. In the last decade the use of social media has given rise to groups who can be from all over the world and help each other out with different research information, treatment options, and cultural supports.

The positive side of online support groups

- Anonymity for members who are uncomfortable discussing their problems in public
- Can offer these people the support they need, often on a twenty-four-hour-a day basis
- People with certain rare diseases who have difficulty pulling together enough people in their area to host group meetings can cover a huge area online, making it easier to find enough people to establish a group
- They offer individuals who are housebound an opportunity to participate in a group

8

CREATE YOUR OASIS

We sometimes grow discouraged
when the things we want to do seem to take
a whole lot longer than we would want them to,
but if there is a goal that must be reached,
on a bridge that would be crossed,
we feel that in the time it takes,
our purposes would all be lost.

But if something is worth doing
then the only thing to do is just a little at a time.

And when you're finally through it,
you will find without a doubt it was far easier
then you imagined, before you started out.

So, if there is a dream that should come,
or a mountain you would climb,
remember that great things are done
just a little at a time.
~ Melanie McDowell. (1974-2006)

This chapter will outline each area of daily living and the strategies and tools I have found helpful to me. I do have to say, my caregiver/ husband performs many of the physical activities in our life. He cannot always be around, as he works full-time to keep us insured, and a part-time job to help give us a little extra money to do some fun positive activities. Like most chronic care families, we run on a tight budget due to medical bills, and the expenses of daily living.

People ask me daily, "How do you do it, How do you do so much?" My key to getting stuff done is to pace myself, know my limits, and be ok with failure when it happens. I am not afraid to fail because I know as long as I am on this earth there is always tomorrow. Every moment is a passing moment. If it is good, cherish it, if it is a challenge, learn from it, and if it is a struggle, remind yourself it too shall pass. I will share the self-care and coping skills that I have learned from my experience to help you live the best life you can, physically and mentally.

The poem at the beginning of this chapter is a great inspiration for me, written by Melanie McDowell. Melanie was my pseudo-stepsister and an RSD sufferer for 12 years. I learned a great deal from her that allowed me to begin my RSD life with encouragement and hope. She is greatly missed, and continues to be an inspiration for me.

I also rely on friends and family to get many things accomplished. I have learned to work when I can and rest when I have to. I know that it is ok to ask for help but not to expect it. Just as I have limitations, those around me do as well, and I have to be respectful of them and myself. Sometimes, this means that I have to prioritize and that not everything on my to-do list will get completed. I had to learn to be ok with this.

It is easy to feel overwhelmed when you live with chronic pain. Every day life can be a struggle, seemingly impossible to overcome. Stay hopeful and take back control of your life. Keep moving forward. Life can still be very enjoyable and you can start with these basic steps:

- A journal to help you become an expert on yourself and your condition

- Accept where you are right now and that you can move forward from here
- Be empowered; focus on the positive side of challenges
- Celebrate your achievements
- Decide what is right for you
- Focus on what makes you feel better
- Just do a little at a time
- Take care of yourself first

Living Well With Chronic Pain

Through our experience in speaking to as many people as we do, if I could give one present to anyone suffering with a chronic condition or chronic pain, it would be hope! Hope keeps you moving forward when everything seems to be pulling you down. Hope will keep the light on at the end of the tunnel. Keep HOPE alive! Take back control of your life by being hopeful. By being hopeful you will move forward and enjoy more moments.

Keep a journal to help you become an expert on yourself and your condition. One of the biggest things I learned is that life can pass you by very quickly and you wake up and wonder where the time went and why you did not do more. Keep track of your surroundings and daily activities. When I started journaling things slowly started to change. One change is that I had to pay attention to days in advance, because what I do today will affect me tomorrow, and the next day.

Accept where you are right now and that you can move forward from here. Embrace your feelings and know that there will be times of sorrow and joy. This is normal in life, but many people facing a chronic condition will begin to focus only on the negative aspects. Remember to pay attention to your starting point each day. Studies show if you start your day with positive thoughts, it helps you through the challenges that arise throughout the day.

This is your life and it is up to you to be empowered. No one else can do this for you. Focus on the positive side of challenges and ask for assistance when needed. Stay socially involved so that you feel a part of something. This is very empowering when you feel as though you have something to offer. Advocate for yourself and others so that you can get the best care possible.

Be flexible to all possibilities but trust yourself when it comes to decisions, like should you have surgery or take a prescribed medication. Do what feels best, not just what others tell you to do. Do not compare yourself to anyone else. Feel proud of whatever you can do. Many times just making it to a doctor's visit is a big accomplishment. Encourage and congratulate yourself as you would a best friend. Celebrating your achievements can be as simple as patting yourself on the back (or wherever it does not hurt).

Take responsibility for meeting your own needs, emotionally, physically, and spiritually. Taking responsibility for yourself does not mean that you have to do it all yourself. Do not feel guilty for needing or asking for help. We cannot all lift heavy objects or push our wheelchair. Decide what is right for you, if that means having to walk slower at least you are still participating.

Prioritize what is most important. Keep track in your journal what activities help you feel better and what makes you worse. Try to avoid the ones that are hard on you. Reorganize your activities or situations to limit your involvement when needed. I am involved in many projects, but I tend to take on projects that do not have a deadline or the deadline is in the far future so that I can be as organized and better able to handle the activity when the time comes. There are times I know if I want to do this event, I must schedule days before and after where all I have to do is rest, so that I will be ready for the event.

Pacing yourself by doing just a little at a time will help you accomplish more in the end. You do not need to get all of the things on your list accomplished in the same day. Prioritize what is needed most and then do the parts you can do when it best fits your energy and activity level.

Be honest with yourself when prioritizing. Ask yourself what makes you feel better, happier, accomplished. How can you achieve these goals? Do you feel guilty or selfish? Remember, the better you feel the better you are. If you need rest every few hours, schedule it in. It is better to take breaks when needed than to push through and hurt yourself. When you take care of yourself emotionally and physically, you are better able to help others. However, if you are not at your best it will be much more difficult to help others to the fullest and you will cause yourself stress. Stay positive and surround yourself with supportive people. Avoid stress, negative people, and complicated situations as much as possible.

Following these steps to your best ability consistently can have positive effect on decreasing your pain and increasing your energy. Your life and health come first and taking positive steps will help you see the difference you are making in your life and accomplishments. Your pain is real but you have control over how you deal with your pain. You should concentrate on just moving in the right direction verses how much you are accomplishing. When others imply that you should be better by now, that you are addicted to your medication, or you are a pessimist, know in your heart that you are doing what you can. This can help you let go of the guilt they are trying to put on you and focus on just feeling the best you can.

Self-Care & Coping Skills

Whether you are in pain or caring for someone in pain, it often seems the weight of the world is on your shoulders. You are worth the investment in yourself! It is easy to send these steps to the backburner but do not let yourself do it. Making the time and energy now can help you feel better and even help you live longer according to studies. In the *Chronic Care in America Survey* done by the Robert Wood Johnson Foundation, in Princeton, New Jersey, people who were organized and made lifestyle changes were more successful at managing their chronic condition than those who did not take the time.[27]

To track your healthcare and be better organized your life it would help to organize your house. Part of the treatment for any chronic condition is lifestyle changes. Here are some things you can do to help combat stress and lighten your responsibilities:

---

[27] Chronic Care in America: a 21st Century Challenge, www.rwjf.org/files/publications/other/ChronicCareinAmerica.pdf

Bedroom

- Blanket support frame so that the weight of blankets or sheets do not rest directly on the feet of a patient
- Install blackout curtains for a place in your house you can retreat to for those moments of breakthrough pain, migraines, etc...
- Keep commonly used items close to the bed for easy reach (remote control, medications, cup of water, reading materials)
- Keep the floor from being cluttered to avoid tripping and falls
- Keep your room ventilated, being too hot or too cold can interfere with quality sleep
- Make sure your mattress is comfortable and use pillows that provide more or less support as needed
- Nightlights in the bedroom and any other rooms where the patient may walk if they awaken during the night

Kitchen

- Come up with easy to make recipes that are still good for you
- Crock pot cooking is a great way to have a good meal and easy to prepare
- Keep commonly used items at waist height, so you don't have to reach
- Large knobs on appliances and cabinet doors requiring manipulation (e.g., stove, dishwasher, washing machine)
- Lightweight dishes and pots such as paper and plastic
- Long handled cleaning appliances, (e.g., brooms, dustpans, sponges)
- Long-handled "grabbers" for removing items on high shelves or picking up items from the floor
- Sliding shelves or turntables on kitchen shelves so the patient does not have to reach into cabinets to access items at the back of a shelf
- Split larger food items or food needing to prepared in Tupperware
- Use electric can and jar openers

Bathroom:

- Dry with smaller towels so the weight of the towel doesn't wear you out or drag across painful areas
- Grab bars in the bathtub, shower, and next to the toilet
- Tub or shower bench
- Use a hairdryer stand
- Use an electric toothbrush
- Use Epsom salt baths to relax

General

- Be as healthy as possible: stop smoking, lose weight, perform you PT exercises, and maintain healthier eating habits
- Electric wheelchair to avoid upper body strain or injury, falls, and add energy to your day
- Keep records organized in binders by provider and then by date
- Know that it is ok if everything is not perfectly clean and tidy
- Medical support professionals and/or accountants to budget for medications, special

appliances, home-nursing care, and other medical-related supplies
- Remove tripping hazards like small rugs
- Use a cordless phone or headset
- Use a digital recorder to keep track of phone conversations and other reminders
- Voice activated lights, appliances, or computer
- Wheelchair access modifications at home

Body
- Check your feet for signs of blisters, cuts, or calluses
- Having a good shoe is important but can mean different things to everyone. For me a flip-flop is best as it is not a tight shoe, can be worn without a sock, and can be slipped on and off easily
- Increase circulation through stretching and light massage
- Keep easy to manage hairstyles
- Try to avoid prolonged pressure on your body. For instance crossing your legs or leaning on your elbows for long periods can cause new

nerve damage due to a lack of blood flow to those areas being compressed

- Visit the dentist and eye doctor at least once a year

Mind

- Complete physical therapy several hours before bedtime
- Concentrate on feelings and ideas that make you feel relaxed
- If something especially stressful is coming up in your life, such as a move or a new job, knowing what you have to do ahead of time can help you cope
- If you are experiencing any emotional issues, you may also find it helpful to talk to a counselor or therapist in addition to your primary care doctor
- If you are not getting enough sleep, it can affect your mood, anxiety levels, ability to cope, and stress levels
- Keeping a daily journal also assists with sleep patterns

- Reducing caffeine intake to help get to sleep and stay asleep longer
- Sleep is important as it helps us avoid health problems and worsening of chronic conditions. A common issue among chronic pain patients is a lack of good sleep
- Write down any thoughts that may wake you up at night so you can put them to rest

Clothing
- Clothes that are wrinkle free, so you do not have to use an iron
- Do laundry in small loads that are lighter and easier to manage
- Flat shoes instead of heels
- Slip-on shoes or velcro instead of shoelaces
- Use clothing that is easy to take on and off that have soft fabrics, avoid buttons, zippers, and complicated outfits

Nutrition
- Cigarette smoking can affect circulation, increasing the risk of foot problems, cancer,

lung issues, and vascular issues. It is also bad
for those around you

- Eat anti-inflammatory foods (dark chocolate,
  fish, garlic, onion, wheatgrass, nuts)
- Go for low-fat meats and dairy products
- Include lots of fruits, vegetables and whole
  grains in your diet

Having Company Over
- Always have an out, so when you want
  company to leave you have a prepared reason
- Have a room in your house that is off limits to
  the guests for you to retreat to when you need a
  break
- Make sure house rules are expressed to
  children (no yelling, fighting, kicking, jumping
  on furniture, etc.)
- Serve snacks that are individualized verses a
  community bowl to keep from passing on
  germs
- Use plastic and paper to serve food and drinks
  to minimize the cleanup effort after company
  leaves

In The Car

- Apply for your handicapped parking placard and keep it in the car
- Car doors that are easy to open and close, keyless entry vehicles and push button start
- Electric seat positions with buttons that are easy to manipulate
- Have the dealership modified controls to facilitate driving
- Keep a pillow and blanket in the car at all times
- Keep an emergency kit in the trunk in at all times (jumper cables, fix a flat, first aid kit)

On A Plane, Train, or Boat

- Arrive early so you can go at a slower, more relaxed pace, this will make the hassles of dealing with disabilities manageable when traveling
- At baggage claim, if you are alone, ask the assistant to get your luggage and to bring you outside to meet your party
- Chew gum or suck on a lifesaver (peppermint, ginger flavors help with nausea) helps balance ear pressure

- Choose a seat on the window or isle based on the parts of your body that are affected so less chance of less bumping into others and having things dropped on you
- Drink water or Gatorade through the flight for hydration
- If possible take an anti-inflammatory medication prior to take off, I've been told it can help with inflammation and lessen the pain of the pressure changes on takeoff and landing
- If traveling alone, bring tip money (one-dollar for each bag that you are assisted with)
- If you are in a wheelchair or scooter, you can skip to the front of the line at security by taking the priority lane. If you need help standing or walking, they will assist you. If you can't be touched due to pain, remember to let the TSA security know prior to them starting their examination
- If you are on oxygen, let the transportation company (airline, train line, or cruise ship) know 30 days prior to travel or as soon as you know that you will be traveling

- If you have any implantation, devices (Portacath, PICC line, Pain Pump, SCS) bring your travel information and a letter from your provider. Allow for extra time at security
- In-flight oxygen needs to be prearranged, and there is typically a charge. Recall 24-48 hours prior to your flight to confirm the oxygen arrangements
- Let the airline personnel know if you need any assistance walking, or an aisle chair to get to your seat
- Let the travel attendant know if you need assistance in using the restroom or need blankets and pillows for comfort
- Let the wheelchair attendant know if you want to make any stops to use the restroom or purchase food while they are assisting you. When they bring you to your gate, ask to be "parked" at the door or the start of the line
- Make sure that the airline person sees you. If you sit off to the side they may miss you and you will not be able to take advantage of pre-boarding

- Once on the plane, if I need to take medication or I am nauseated, I ask for a small glass of water
- Pack your medications in a carry-on bag. If your luggage gets lost, you will not have to worry about where or how to get your medications
- Plan ahead with the internet to get destination information
- Request handicapped services from the airline, bus depot, car rental company, and hotel all ahead of time
- When parking, use your phone to take a picture of the area you parked in so when you return it is easy to find
- When you arrive at your destination, stay in your seat until your wheelchair assistance has arrived. They typically ask you to wait until the other passengers unload so that you do not hold them up or so that they do not bump against you and cause you further injury

Make the Most of Your Medical Visits

- Be assertive and listen to the other side
- Become the expert of your pain. Increasing your communication leads to better treatment and pain relief
- Better communication begins with organization. Start a pain journal
- Bring a list of all the medications— prescription, over-the-counter, and herbal— that you take
- Have a shared understanding of goals
- Identify your top concerns, questions, and symptoms
- Learning to communicate with your healthcare professionals is important in your treatment plan
- Schedule your appointment at the end of the day. If you have the last appointment, your provider may not feel as rushed to get through your visit in order to get to the next patient
- Take responsibility to reach the goals

During Your Medical Visit

- Communicate what has happened to you medically since your last visit
- Describe what your pain feels like: burning, cutting, stabbing, deep, tingling, etc. Different types of pain can be treated with different medications. Be as descriptive as possible for a better outcome with pain relief
- Express what makes pain better/worse - it helps to keep a journal
- How does the pain affect your daily living: do you need help dressing, bathing, or cooking
- If you are unclear about what your provider has told you, double check by repeating what you think you heard. "I think what I heard you say is XYZ, is that what you meant?"
- It is also important to keep your emotions under control
- It is important that you stay on track and focused at your doctor appointments
- Keep follow up appointments
- Life stressors and anxiety can worsen pain symptoms, so be sure to tell your provider if you feel depressed or unusually anxious

- State what concerns or worries you have regarding the pain, medications; e.g., what if the pain just does not go away
- Take a minute to remind your provider of important things in your medical history. If your medical history is complicated, bring your medical records with you to save time
- Take notes during the visit or consider asking a trusted friend or family member to accompany you
- The more you are prepared and on track the better your care will be

Protecting Prescription Medications
- Do not request early refills or increase your dose of medication without discussing it with your provider
- Keep medications out of reach of children and pets, and use child proof caps
- Keep prescription medications away from teenagers and visiting guests (friends and family members have also been known to steal prescription drugs)

- Lost or stolen opioid medications are a red flag for possible abuse [28]
- Open the container over a counter, away from the sink or toilet
- Participate in a drug-monitoring program such as the Patient Physician Trust Partnership. www.pptp.org
- Protect your supply as you would guard other valuables, such as a box with a combination lock
- The best place to store your medicine is in a cool, dry place in its original container. Most medications lose their effectiveness in warm, moist areas
- The goal of medication is improved function. Keep track in your journal, what you are able to do because of relief you are receiving from the medication and any side effects that you develop; be sure to communicate this to your provider

---

[28] Protecting your prescriptions, Lost or stolen opioid medications are a red flag for possible abuse, Bill McCarberg, MD, and Maggie Buckley, APF Bd. Member; APF's Pain Community News, Winter 2008, Volume 8

DEDICATION

For 10 years now I have been living the life of a chronic pain patient navigating the health system. In the beginning, I did a poor job. We are not taught growing up how to be our own best advocates, patient rights, or that we have a stake in our health. I know now we need to act deliberately and responsibly. This book came about after a discussion with a patient and friend, Melissa Lucero. One of my life goals is to provide a guide map through the system for other patients and their families. With one in three people having a chronic condition that causes pain, you or someone you know is affected.

I hope that the readers find use in the topics and details I have shared. I have combined what I have learned personally with resources I have created or gathered to help you walk through the minefield of the health system without hitting a mine. The title of the book was the concept of another patient and friend, Kyle Kendrix. Kyle has been a go to friend for me as he has had Reflex Sympathetic Dystrophy (RSD), the same condition as me, for longer than I have. He has tried treatment options that I have not and he is able to support me in making decisions for my own care.

These past few months we have had many losses in Pain Community. Michelle Malone, Dec. 18, 2011 (RSD), Adriana Catherine Biba, April 26, 2012 (RSD), Danielle Freudenheim, May 5, 2012

(RSD), Debbie Fellows, June 30, 2012 (RSD) and too many others. May God bless their souls and give peace to their family and friends.

My great friend Danielle will be especially missed by my husband and me. We miss her but we know she is in a better place and is now pain free. I think of her kindness, friendship, and support on a daily basis. She was always there for me and I know she will be shining a light on my life from heaven. I remember her as a cheerleader of hope for me and how happy she was after one particular treatment from Dr. Sims. He was able to provide her some relief and give her a tool so that she was able to get out and do more before she passed away. My happy memories of her carry me through this sorrowful time.

Many Blessings!
Barby Ingle

Find Barby Online
www.barbyingle.com
www.faceboo.com/rsdinme
www.facebook.com/barby.ingle
www.facebook.com/barbyingleauthor
www.facebook.com/remissionpossible
www.facebook.com/thepaincode
www.linkedin.com/barby.ingle
www.twitter.com/barby.ingle
www.youtube.com/barbyallyn

Other Books by Barby Ingle

Barby's books are for all of those suffering from chronic pain as well as their family, caregivers, healthcare professionals and public. Until you feel the pain, it is difficult to understand the challenges it brings on even after remission is successfully reached. Her books put this into great perspective with easy to follow and understand information.

Whether a person is dealing with physical or mental pain, it can and will consume you if you allow it to. Only the patient can begin the process of healing, and Barby's hope is that these books will inspire the patient's eventual transformation filled with HOPE. Healing starts from within and it is "Yours If You Choose to Accept It".

The Pain Code; Workbook and Journal

When it comes to living, the best life you can when faced with a chronic care condition every person has choices. It is a matter of finding the right fit for you. The patient can either let the disease run them or sort through the system and take control of the disease. Coping with a chronic condition takes hope and self-awareness. This workbook and journal will help you discover how to talk with your providers, includes sample insurance company letters and organizational information so you can become your own best advocate. Getting organized is very important. It will take work in the beginning but it gets easier as you go. You can also save yourself more pain and challenges down the road by being organized with your approach to treating your chronic medical issue.

RSD in Me! A Patient and Caregivers Guide to RSD and Other Chronic Pain Conditions goes through aspects of Reflex Sympathetic Dystrophy Syndrome (RSD/CRPS) and chronic pain including definition, causes, tips on dealing with healthcare professionals, emotional aspects, caretaker information, of dealing with chronic pain and tips on coping with the pain. The Executive Director of the Power of Pain Foundation wrote this book as a pain patient, based on personal experiences in dealing with pain and the healthcare system. Barby earned a degree in Social Psychology in 1994 from George Mason University. She worked as a Division IA Collegiate head coach at Washington State University for eight years and was a successful business owner until an auto accident in 2002. Topics cover a wide range from history of RSD, causes, symptoms, diagnosing, psychosocial aspects, patient's perspective, treatment plans, change in family dynamics, spirituality when in pain, working with the healthcare industry, helpful tips to use every day and more. This book has been over six years in the making. A pain patient writes it from her perspective of the health system. This book will touch the lives of many patients. Proceeds raised from the sale of this book go to the funding of patient grants and awareness projects for the foundation.

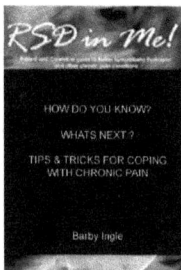

ReMission Possible; Yours, If You Chose to Accept It is a valuable look into the process of healing socially, emotionally and physically after remission is achieved. Life does not just go back to the way it was before your illness. Recognizing this and moving through it can help you adjust to the new life that you now face. This book is about a patient's journey, (one year leading up to an IV-Infusion treatment that put author Barby Ingle into remission and one year of what happened after) of health, social; and mental adjustments. *ReMission Possible* is a follow up book to *RSD in Me* but also stands alone as a story that you too can achieve. It is a motivational guide to being your own best advocate, "The Chief of Staff of Your Own Medical Team" as Barby likes to say. All of Barby Ingle's books are wide reaching with one in three Americans dealing with a chronic pain condition of some sort.

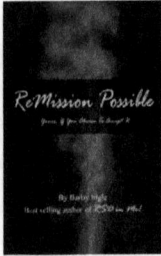